THE OPIOID FIX

THE OPIOID FIX

AMERICA'S ADDICTION CRISIS AND THE SOLUTION THEY DON'T WANT YOU TO HAVE

BARBARA ANDRAKA-CHRISTOU

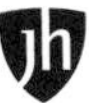

JOHNS HOPKINS UNIVERSITY PRESS
Baltimore

Printed in the United States of America on acid-free paper
9 8 7 6 5 4 3 2 1

Johns Hopkins University Press
2715 North Charles Street
Baltimore, Maryland 21218-4363
www.press.jhu.edu

Library of Congress Cataloging-in-Publication Data

Names: Andraka-Christou, Barbara, 1988– author.
Title: The opioid fix : America's addiction crisis and the solution they don't want you to have / Barbara Andraka-Christou.
Description: Baltimore : Johns Hopkins University Press, 2020. | Includes bibliographical references and index.
Identifiers: LCCN 2019028033 | ISBN 9781421437651 (hardcover ; alk. paper) | ISBN 9781421437668 (ebook)
Subjects: MESH: Opioid-Related Disorders—drug therapy | Opiate Substitution Treatment | Health Policy | Opioid-Related Disorders—epidemiology | United States—epidemiology
Classification: LCC RC568.O45 | NLM WM 284 | DDC 362.29/3—dc23
LC record available at https://lccn.loc.gov/2019028033

A catalog record for this book is available from the British Library.

Special discounts are available for bulk purchases of this book. For more information, please contact Special Sales at specialsales@press.jhu.edu.

Johns Hopkins University Press uses environmentally friendly book materials, including recycled text paper that is composed of at least 30 percent post-consumer waste, whenever possible.

To the dozens of courageous people recovering from opioid addiction who have shared their stories with me

And to my husband, Alex, who has supported all my dreams

The best time to plant a tree was 20 years ago.
The second-best time is now.

CHINESE PROVERB

Contents

THE OPIOID FIX

INTRODUCTION

"DO YOU THINK YOU CAN handle the whole story? Or do you want the PG version?" Jackson asked me over the phone.*

"Just tell me as much or as little as you feel comfortable sharing," I responded.

By now I have heard many gritty stories of opioid addiction, which is the compulsive use of opioids despite negative consequences. For the past three years I have spent a significant portion of my time interviewing people in recovery, their families, health care providers, criminal justice system employees, and policy makers. I have conducted more than 120 in-depth interviews and analyzed hundreds of hours of interview transcripts. Not to mention the numerous informal discussions with concerned people, ranging from police officers to twelve-step group leaders to other public health researchers like me.

I wish I could say that the story Jackson went on to tell me was an anomaly—that few Americans experience the kind of early childhood trauma he faced prior to regularly misusing drugs. But according to a world-famous series of studies on adverse childhood experiences,

* All interviewee names, including names of health care providers and judges in chapters 5 and 6, have been changed. Additionally, certain details of their stories, such as specific locations, dates, and professions, have been changed to protect their confidentiality. See the last section of this chapter for more information about my methodology.

drug use and drug addiction are strongly predicted by trauma during childhood. These events range from sexual assault to emotional abuse to physical battery and neglect. According to one of the most cited peer-reviewed medical studies on the topic, two-thirds of injection drug use is attributable to childhood abuse or trauma.[1] The initial adverse childhood experiences study, which involved seventeen thousand participants, mostly white, middle-class individuals with health insurance, found a "dose-response" relationship between trauma and substance use disorder.[2] In other words, the greater the trauma, the more intense the substance use disorder. Since that first study, numerous other studies have found similar results in a wide variety of populations.[3]

From a scientific standpoint, the relationship between adverse childhood experiences and addiction is unsurprising for two reasons. First, adverse childhood events may cause mental illness, such as post-traumatic stress disorder, anxiety disorder, or depression, and people with mental illness may self-medicate with drugs,[4] especially if they have not learned positive coping strategies.[5] Children raised in harmful or unsupportive homes are less likely than those raised in supportive homes to learn healthy ways of modulating their emotions.[5] Second, trauma negatively impacts the parts of the brain, neurological pathways, and behaviors that are implicated in substance use disorders. For example, trauma may increase impulsivity, and impulsivity may increase the likelihood of using drugs.[6]

For many people, drugs become a coping mechanism for post-traumatic stress disorder or depression. Others experience opioid addiction after repeated exposure to prescription pain medications, such as oxycodone or hydrocodone, following an injury. The latter is called *iatrogenic* addiction, meaning caused by medical treatment. In the past two decades, the number of opioid prescriptions written by physicians quadrupled for conditions such as chronic pain. This increase reflected a response to unethical marketing by pharmaceutical companies and pressure from the US government to alleviate patients' pain.[7] Not surprisingly, iatrogenic addiction quadrupled during that same time period.[7]

The United States is facing a health crisis in which more than 115 Americans die daily from opioid overdoses,[8] with 500,000 deaths expected in the next decade. The crisis is a result of both supply and demand forces. On the demand side, many people initially exposed to opioids for pain management developed an addiction to opioids, and numerous people with untreated mental health disorders sought opioids as self-medication. On the supply side, opioids became widely available, due to both the overprescribing of opioids for pain management and an influx of readily available, cheap heroin and illicit fentanyl as substitutes.[9] Prescription pain medications, opium, heroin, and fentanyl are all opioids and affect the brain in essentially the same way.

Despite the media's focus on upper-middle-class families exposed to Oxycontin following an injury, most people whom I have interviewed come from a lower socioeconomic background, often with parents struggling with their own addiction, unemployment, or mental health issues. Opioid addiction is often called an "equal opportunity" problem because it can affect anyone of any background. According to the National Institute on Drug Abuse, however, such terminology obscures the fact that the hardest hit populations have been those from lower socioeconomic backgrounds as well as people in rural areas, such as Appalachia.[10] A stressful environment, such as one with limited employment opportunities, negatively impacts mental health, increasing the likelihood that an individual will develop a substance use disorder.[10] Combine such social disparity with untreated mental health disorders and an influx of opioids and you've got a full-blown public health crisis.

Regardless of how addiction starts, the National Institute on Drug Abuse and other scientific institutions call opioid addiction a biopsychosocial brain disease.[11] In other words, it is caused by a complex combination of biological, psychological, and social factors.

Many other less stigmatized chronic diseases likewise result from these factors, including diabetes, depression, chronic hypertension, and asthma.

Jackson's story is one of the more harrowing ones I've heard. It really starts with his mother's story, as do many narratives of multigenerational drug addiction. Jackson's mother, Kelly, was a victim of incest, repeatedly raped by her father in a small Midwestern town in 1970s America, a time when police preferred to look the other way and stay out of "family matters." At the age of fifteen, she gave birth to Jackson. By then she was already using crack cocaine.

When she was pregnant with Jackson, Kelly moved in with her boyfriend, though the relationship was neither healthy nor stable. The boyfriend also used crack cocaine, along with alcohol and marijuana. Jackson's first memory of drugs was at the age of three. His mom was throwing a party in their rundown apartment. Lines of cocaine lay ready for snorting on the living room coffee table. Seeking refuge, Jackson climbed over passed-out bodies on the living room floor to reach his mother. Kelly grabbed him and forced a marijuana joint in his mouth, clamping his nose with her fingers, while her friends looked on and laughed at the three-year-old getting high. Jackson's mother then poured an entire bottle of beer into his mouth, with more laughter ensuing. It's not hard to understand why Jackson was regularly smoking marijuana and drinking by the age of seven.

When he was six years old, Jackson was raped for the first time. It was his next-door neighbor, who was also his babysitter. Kelly found her son sobbing later that evening. After Jackson told her what the neighbor had done, she marched over to the neighbor's house demanding an explanation and an apology. She got what she wanted, and the neighbor promised to never rape Jackson again. The next time Jackson's mother went out and needed a babysitter, she hired the same neighbor.

By the age of ten, Jackson was so neglected that the state's Department of Child Services took him away and placed him with a foster family. That family was okay—stable but not particularly kind toward the melancholy boy who would sometimes start shaking for no reason. But as often happens to foster children, Jackson was eventually sent to a new family. This family had a blond man who asked Jackson to call him "Dad." Then, like the old next-door neighbor, "Dad" proceeded to regularly sexually assault Jackson. So, Jackson ran away.

By fifteen, Jackson's "home" consisted of homeless shelters or friends' sofas. He was also using every drug he could get his hands on. He had never been to a counselor, let alone a dentist. He hated his life, regularly skipped school, and felt miserable. More than once he thought of killing himself. Arguably, the best thing that ever happened to him was when his girlfriend, Diana, got pregnant at the age of seventeen.

Jackson wanted to be a good father. But he knew this meant not getting high every day or else the Department of Child Services would take his daughter away too, just like they had taken him away from his mother. He'd only ever heard of one resource to stop using drugs: Alcoholics Anonymous (AA). It was also the only recovery method available in his small city. Jackson started attending AA meetings regularly and, for the first time in his life, associated with older men who were not abusive, who did not use drugs, and who seemed to have his best interests at heart. It was like having multiple father figures. Jackson could call his sponsor at all hours, and the sponsor, a selfless, caring middle-aged man, would take Jackson out for a cup of coffee and talk.

Having dropped out of high school along with his girlfriend, Jackson worked odd jobs, mainly in the fast-food industry, to support his young family. But the local fast-food restaurants were flooded with drugs. The local heroin dealer was his coworker. And Jackson, who had still never received any counseling or psychiatric medication, had undiagnosed post-traumatic stress disorder, or PTSD. Almost every night he had nightmares. Sometimes he didn't want to get out of bed in the morning, hoping to die instead. Heroin, more than anything, made him feel better. It numbed his emotions and gave him a sense of temporary internal peace—until he would experience severe withdrawal symptoms (diarrhea, vomiting, shaking, muscle spasms, and itching) coupled with profound cravings for more drugs. Despite AA and the support of his sponsor, Jackson's heroin use escalated as he became tolerant to lower doses. He shifted from snorting to injecting heroin so it would have a stronger, faster effect.

When Jackson's daughter was a toddler, Jackson and Diana broke up. They had never had much in common other than drug use. Diana was in rehab and Jackson was basically homeless, so his daughter moved in with Diana's mother, someone with whom Jackson had always had a poor relationship. Diana's mother prevented Jackson from seeing his own daughter more than a few times per month because of his drug use—which was ironic since Diana's mother seemed to have a drinking problem and Diana herself went in and out of rehab.

Jackson's life seemed to stand still even though he was aging. He loved his daughter and wanted to be the stable father figure he had never had. But each time he stopped heroin, he would feel depressed and relapse again. It was a vicious cycle of attending AA meetings, followed by internal promises to start on the path of recovery, followed by cravings and withdrawals, followed by depression and eventually relapse. Ten years passed, and he was still working in the fast-food industry. His social network bounced back and forth between the AA group and drug users, depending on whether he was using.

At one point, his AA sponsor, who had long suspected Jackson had PTSD, suggested that Jackson see a counselor. He had no health insurance, something food industry jobs rarely provide, but fortunately he found a public mental health clinic with payments based on a sliding scale of income. The counselor had training in both mental health and substance use disorders and was devoted to her work. But dredging up the painful memories made him want to escape into drugs even more. After every session, he felt so overwhelmed with toxic memories that it took all his courage to avoid heroin. Sometimes, the heroin won. After a few weeks, Jackson quit counseling.

Then something fortuitous occurred. Jackson asked his "friend," Ryan, to bring him heroin. Ryan explained that he was no longer shooting up. He was trying to quit with the help of a medication-assisted treatment, or MAT, called Suboxone. He was buying Suboxone off the street since he could not find an actual doctor to prescribe it. Ryan would take Suboxone a few times a day, which would prevent him from getting high by blocking heroin's effects. Plus, Suboxone took away cravings for heroin and prevented withdrawal symptoms. The craziest part was that it did not make him high, it just made him feel normal, even though Suboxone activates the brain's opioid receptors.[12] Suboxone is an opioid but it acts differently than other opioids.

Jackson was interested in this new medication. After all, he had tried counseling and AA. He could not afford rehab. Furthermore, all his friends who went to rehab started using again as soon as they got out. So like Ryan, he started buying Suboxone off the street. Without a doctor, though, it was hard to figure out exactly how much to take to prevent withdrawals and cravings. If he took too little, the Suboxone was worthless. If he took too much, it was a waste of money because Suboxone has something called a "ceiling effect," wherein after a certain point, any additional Suboxone has no impact on the brain. And Suboxone was expensive, more so than other things sold on the street at the time. But as Ryan had predicted, the Suboxone took away most of Jackson's cravings for heroin. And even if a fleeting heroin craving did occur, the knowledge that the Suboxone in his system would prevent a heroin high stopped him from shooting up.

Jackson, who was trying to avoid the drug-dealing streets as much as possible, searched for a Suboxone-prescribing doctor. But none existed within a one-hundred-mile radius of his city. He started driving out of town once each month to see a physician who would prescribe a thirty-day supply picked up from a drugstore on the condition that

Jackson visit a counselor monthly. Sometimes when his car was out of commission or he lacked gas money, Jackson would pay others to drive him to the doctor. Sometimes the payment consisted of giving them some of his paper-thin Suboxone strips. They reminded him of mouthwash strips, dissolving in your mouth after a few minutes but less tasty, with an orange flavor that sometimes made him a little queasy.

Complying with the doctor's orders, Jackson found a new mental health counselor at the same public health center he had once attended. The counselor signed a monthly form to confirm that Jackson was going to his appointments and then faxed it to the doctor's office. The counselor always seemed annoyed with the paperwork and the fact that Jackson was getting Suboxone. Even though a large percentage of the treatment center's patients had opioid problems, the center did not provide Suboxone, and Jackson felt that any discussions about the medication seemed awkward and inappropriate.

Jackson's new counselor reaffirmed the first counselor's diagnosis of PTSD. Treatment included processing painful experiences, realizing that he was not at fault for the abuse he had suffered, and adopting new coping mechanisms. Even though Suboxone had no direct effect on the PTSD, it gave him the physiological stability to do the psychological work. It was incredibly difficult: "The hardest work I've ever done," Jackson told me over the phone. "And I'm still working through [the memories]."

The counseling sessions were excruciating, usually ending in a flood of tears and shaking, something he used to do as a kid. Even if Jackson wanted the temporary peaceful reprieve of heroin, he knew it would be a waste of money with Suboxone in his system. So instead, after a particularly hard session, he would call his AA sponsor or watch TV. And most days when he was not in a counseling session, Jackson had few or no cravings. For once, he could focus energy on reuniting with his daughter and, eventually, finding a new job.

Today Jackson is a peer recovery coach. That means he works for an addiction treatment center as a kind of guide for those who are just starting their recovery processes. He still takes Suboxone daily, though at a lower dosage than when he began the medication. Eventually, he plans to switch to another medication, called Vivitrol, which would block opioid effects without activating the opioid receptors. But it would take a two-week detoxification process, which could be destabilizing. Jackson doesn't think there is any real need for him to get off the Suboxone; it has been working well for years with few side effects. But he worries that someone at the treatment center will learn of his Suboxone therapy. He knows of other staff who were fired for having Suboxone appear in their employee urine drug screens. Since Vivitrol doesn't activate the opioid receptors like Suboxone does, it might be a more accepted treatment option.

I ask if he sees any signs of change, if people are becoming more open to the idea of Suboxone or MAT in general. He replies that he hasn't seen many signs of change in his local recovery community. In fact, Jackson is more concerned about revealing his Suboxone treatment status than his history of heroin addiction: "I don't feel like there's enough people right now that view MAT as a legitimate treatment. I think that we're starting to see it go that direction, but there's enough of that stigma still left that I'm just too afraid to be open about that . . . It's kind of like in the nineties, there was still gay-bashing going on, but for the most part people accepted that there were gay people. It wasn't the fifties, right? But it was still too scary to come out in high school. It's the same kind of stigma. I don't feel like this is the time yet for someone who's on MAT who works in the field to feel 100 percent safe to say, 'I'm on MAT.' You know what I mean?"

It's been over fifteen years since Suboxone was approved by the US Food and Drug Administration (FDA), and the treatment center where Jackson works still harbors the antiquated, misguided view that Suboxone is a sign of personal failure and just another drug of abuse. And it's not just the treatment center that silences him. Jackson continues to attend AA almost daily, but no one there knows he takes Suboxone either. Why not, I ask? "Because they would think I'm a fake. That I'm not really sober."

I find this profoundly unfair. Jackson has not touched an illegal drug or misused a legal medication in over three years. He has a job. He finally has shared custody of his daughter, the love of his life. He is afraid to tell people in the recovery community about one of the most important tools in his recovery, even though his job is to guide others on their recovery journeys. It is a common fear that I have heard again and again during my interviews. People who have worked so hard to manage their addiction in the face of insurmountable odds (poverty, trauma, mental health issues), and have triumphed despite these obstacles, keep their stories hidden.

PEER-REVIEWED STUDY after peer-reviewed study shows that medications such as Suboxone and methadone are the most reliable and most effective treatment for opioid addiction.[14] They cut the rate of death from overdose in half[14] because people stop taking dangerous amounts of heroin or prescription pain medicines. They prevent the spread of HIV/AIDS, hepatitis C, and other communicable diseases because people stop injecting drugs and sharing the needles.[15–17] Medication helps decrease criminal activity[18] and increase employment rates and social functioning.[19]

Yet more than 60 percent of US addiction treatment centers fail to provide any FDA-approved medications for treating opioid addiction, sometimes even barring entry to those taking the medications Suboxone or methadone.[20,21] Abstinence-only treatment—treatment that explicitly denies the validity and place of medications in managing addiction—is the norm.

This is not to disparage counseling or support groups, such as AA, upon which abstinence-only treatment centers typically depend. Counseling and support groups are critical for addressing underlying psychological and social issues, as they have been in Jackson's case. But counseling and support groups, collectively called "psychosocial" or "behavioral" treatments, are less likely to address physiological cravings and withdrawal symptoms or prevent the ability to get high. That is why a meta-analysis of studies by Cochrane, a highly regarded medical research organization, has definitively stated that medications for treating addiction are more effective than behavioral treatment alone at preventing relapse and overdose,[13,22] though in many cases, behavioral and pharmacological treatment should be combined.[23] It's why the World Health Organization urges every country to provide low-cost medications for treating addiction within prisons and jails,[24,25] calling buprenorphine and methadone "essential medicines." It's why the US government through the National Institute on Drug Abuse, the Substance Abuse and Mental Health Services Administration, and the Food and Drug Administration urges the expansion of medications in opioid addiction treatment.[11,23,26] The US surgeon general has called the combination of medications and psychosocial treatment the "gold standard" for opioid addiction.[27] After an in-depth review of the evidence, the National Academies of Sciences, Engineering, and Medicine released a statement in 2019 titled *Medications for Opioid Use Disorder Save Lives*, in which they maintain that withholding MAT for any reason in any facility is unethical.[28] Additionally, the National Academies explicitly states that allowing only one form of MAT, such as extended-release naltrexone (i.e., Vivitrol), while forbidding other forms, such as buprenorphine (i.e., Suboxone) or methadone, is unethical.[28]

What is a successful addiction treatment program? After reviewing hundreds of peer-reviewed studies in medicine and public health and analyzing over 120 interviews, I believe the following:

A successful addiction treatment program is one that offers a wide range of evidence-based treatments backed by rigorous scientific studies, without unnecessary legal and institutional barriers, without stigma, in a client-centric manner.

In other words, addiction should be treated the way we treat other chronic medical conditions with biological, psychological, and social components, such as hypertension or depression.

In 2016 alone, the opioid crisis claimed more American lives than were claimed by the entire Vietnam War,[29] and it decreased the average US life expectancy.[30] Yet opioid addiction's most effective treatment is heavily stigmatized, from physicians' offices, to counselors' offices and rehabilitation centers, to prisons and jails and drug courts. Perhaps most shockingly, medication-related stigma comes from the recovery community too, including within support groups like AA, which frequently tell people medication means "you are not really sober," "you are just using a crutch," or "you're just replacing one addiction with another"—even if the person has not misused opioids for years.

My initial purpose in writing this book was twofold: to examine the historical, legal, and cultural reasons for limited use of medications in addiction treatment and to identify potential policy solutions to this problem. But over time I have adopted a third purpose: to validate the experience of the hundreds of thousands of Americans who have often secretly undergone recovery from opioid addiction with the help of medication. Their experiences show that US addiction treatment is frequently not based on the latest scientific evidence and is rarely person-centered. Addiction is a chronic medical condition that is still treated in an unscientific manner and outside of mainstream medicine.

LIKE MOST RESEARCHERS, my work is informed by a variety of theoretical frameworks that guide interpretation of what might otherwise be a sea of incongruous data. Specifically, I use the socio-ecological model of health services to understand health services barriers and facilitators identified by interviewees. According to this model, there are four levels of factors that can either push or pull an individual toward treatment.[31] Each of these levels is independently important, but they also interact. They help explain how an effective treatment, such as medication, can exist but be grossly underutilized.

The first level is the individual level, which includes a person's health and social history, demographics, beliefs, values, and behaviors. For example, a female with a history of domestic violence may find it difficult to share her recovery story in a counseling group filled with men. If she has a low income, she may forgo treatment simply because she cannot afford it. If she believes that a certain treatment is ineffective or socially stigmatized, she may not even consider it.

The next level, the relationship level, presumes that one's inner circle of relationships, such as friends and family, affect whether one seeks and complies with treatment. For example, someone in a relationship with an active drug user may find it difficult to stick with a treatment method when constantly faced with drug use "triggers" pulling him or her back toward drug use. Alternatively, relationships can propel someone toward treatment. In Jackson's story, it was his relationship with Ryan that ultimately propelled him toward treatment with a medication.

The third level, community, includes local resources and institutions, such as the availability of treatment providers in the city. Obviously, even if one is highly motivated to begin treatment and lives in a supportive household, the lack of any local treatment provider will prove a huge deterrent to compliance. Not finding a provider can be very discouraging, undermining motivation for treatment.

Finally, the fourth level is the societal or policy level, which includes such factors as laws and the broader culture. Laws impact the availability of community resources, including methadone clinics and buprenorphine treatment providers. Likewise, culture affects whether a person seeks treatment and then whether he or she sticks with treatment. For example, the antimedication attitudes associated with the twelve-step support movement may deter people from sticking with buprenorphine or methadone treatment as they experience pressure from group members to quit. Finally, laws and culture interact. Laws are informed by cultural assumptions about drug users, including that they are dangerous and should be locked up rather than treated. Cultural assumptions are likewise informed by laws, especially criminal laws that make it seem like drug users are immoral simply because they are doing something illegal.

My work is also informed by the theory of reasoned action and planned behavior.[32] This theory is particularly applicable to the first level of the socio-ecological model: the individual level. The theory has been validated in the substance use disorder treatment context and assumes that people's intention to seek treatment or stick with treatment is predicted by three constructs:

1. A person's beliefs about the treatment, such as whether the treatment will help solve a problem;
2. Perceptions of social norms surrounding the treatment, such as whether others view the treatment positively; and
3. Feelings of self-efficacy, such as whether one can really do the treatment (e.g., whether one has the financial means or the necessary transportation).

The theory likewise applies to health care providers. For example, if physicians think buprenorphine is dangerous, feel social pressure from colleagues *against* prescribing buprenorphine, and worry that they lack adequate training, they are unlikely to prescribe buprenorphine to patients.

These theoretical frameworks are important because they help explain why the mere existence of an effective treatment, even one that lowers the risk of death from overdose by approximately 50 percent, is rarely prescribed or used.[14] Clearly, it is insufficient for a lifesaving drug to merely exist in the market; it may still never be accessed. Treatment occurs not in a vacuum but in a complex legal and cultural context with multiple levels of potential barriers and facilitators to retention and compliance. The job of health service researchers such as myself is to tease out health service barriers and facilitators so that micro and macro level policies can be created to address them.

In my research I rely heavily on interviews with a variety of people who have an effect on, provide, or use health services for addiction, including current drug users, people in recovery, their family members, activists, criminal justice professionals, policy makers, and health care providers. In-depth interviews, especially unstructured or semistructured interviews, allow me to explore a wide range of experiences without established preconceptions. Even though I approach interviews with questions in hand, often new topics emerge that I had not anticipated as I prepared for the interview. In a poorly understood research area involving vulnerable social groups, such openness in methodology is an asset. My interviews have led me to venture into new areas of research that I had previously not considered.

After my interviews are professionally transcribed, I analyze them for themes in collaboration with other researchers. I typically use an approach called "thematic analysis," wherein we apply "codes" to topics that seem to repeatedly appear across interviews. These codes are basically like different-colored highlighters but are applied in a software package called Dedoose. My research team members and I independently code topics in each transcript and then compare our results, discussing and negotiating any differences. Since qualitative research can be subjective, this process, called "consensus coding," helps ensure that I am not seeing something in the data that is not there. For example, I might read a quotation in an interview transcript that I think means the interviewee distrusts his physician, so I code it as "physician distrust"; but my colleague may not see physician distrust in this quotation at all. After comparing our codes, we negotiate and come to an agreement about the final application of the code.

After completing the consensus coding process, the research team then views all transcript excerpts associated with a certain code.

For instance, we might pull all excerpts coded as "physician distrust" from all interviews. After reading and rereading these excerpts, we identify patterns within and across codes. We might, for example, find that interviewees who feel stigmatized by their physicians are the ones who distrust their physicians' motivations. In the end, we call this observation a "theme."

The purpose of qualitative research, such as interview data collection and analysis, is not to identify frequencies (e.g., 50 percent of drug users have tried buprenorphine treatment), because the sampling is not representative. Often when I interview people who use drugs, the sampling is not even random but rather "snowball," meaning that I start with a group of drug users or people in recovery who then connect me to their friends, who connect me to their friends, and so forth. It is a well-respected method for reaching stigmatized populations who often prefer to remain secret.

Instead, the purpose of qualitative research is largely exploratory, to identify themes in the population sampled. These themes can later inform quantitative methods, such as surveys, which can provide a representative, random sample of opinions and experiences. But the first exploratory step is very important, because without it we might not even know what questions to ask in a survey. After all, a survey, unlike a semistructured or unstructured interview, is primarily composed of close-ended questions wherein the researcher guesses and provides potential survey answers ahead of time. The other benefit of qualitative research is that the data is "rich," illuminating the context and relationships between different actors, cultures, and policies. Qualitative data allows one to paint a picture in a way that many quantitative methods rarely permit, given their topic and answer-choice restrictions.

Rich qualitative data complements quantitative data, suggesting potential reasons why a phenomenon is occurring. For example, quantitative analysis of deidentified electronic health records demonstrates that medication-assisted treatment retention rates are frustratingly low. But why are people dropping out of treatment? By interviewing these people and hearing their stories, we can learn about the barriers they face as well as hear their perspectives on what might lead them to stick with treatment. Such data is not available in the electronic health record but can help policy makers create tailored policies that directly address the problem. I hope that my research helps you, the reader, better understand the results from quantitative studies in a rich context of individual, interpersonal, community, and societal layers impacting health services.

All interviewee names, including those of the judges and health care providers in chapters 5 and 6, have been changed. Certain details of their stories, too, such as specific locations, dates, and professions, have sometimes been changed to protect their confidentiality. For interviewees in recovery, sometimes I have combined two stories into one story to further ensure confidentiality and to ease readability. For example, I may combine John Doe's story of how he started misusing opioids with Jane Doe's opioid addiction treatment experience. Additionally, based on my experience of visiting treatment centers and support group meetings, I provide sensory details to assist you in having a fuller picture. For example, I may not have attended John's specific AA meeting, but I have seen enough of them to know it was likely in a church basement with people seated in a circle, the smell of inexpensive coffee filling the room, and AA brochures and books distributed on empty chairs. Otherwise, all the stories you will read are true and the quotes are taken verbatim from interviews.

Interviews were conducted between 2015 and 2019, with the majority of participants coming from Indiana or Florida due to my physical presence in these two states, though in total interviewees came from thirteen states. Of the 120-plus interviews I have conducted, about sixty have been with individuals recovering from a substance use disorder. Approximately four dozen of these interviewees were recovering from opioid addiction. Among those interviewees, approximately 90 percent had experience with MAT, 90 percent had experience with twelve-step support groups, and two-thirds had experience with residential rehabilitation. Approximately half were male and half were female, with the vast majority of both groups being white, non-Hispanic. Their ages ranged from young adult to upper sixties.

Finally, a few comments on terminology. The *Diagnostic and Statistical Manual of Mental Disorders*, essentially the bible of mental health treatment, recently changed and no longer uses the term *opioid addiction*, preferring *opioid use disorder* instead. I have purposely chosen to continue using *opioid addiction* in this book because it is essentially a severe form of opioid use disorder, and the focus of this book is on people with moderate to severe opioid use disorder, not on people who occasionally misuse opioids. It is also a lot easier to write "opioid addiction" than "moderate or severe opioid use disorder."

I have also struggled with whether to use the phrase "medication-assisted treatment" or the more modern terms "pharmacotherapy" or "medications for opioid use disorder" instead. Ultimately, I have chosen "medication-assisted treatment" because it remains the dominant term used to refer to FDA-approved medications for treating opioid addiction, such as methadone, buprenorphine, and naltrexone. With that said, "medication-assisted treatment" is an imperfect term because it incorrectly implies that medication is not enough of a treatment—that it just "assists" treatment—though for many people it is the only tool needed for recovery. Technically speaking, MAT refers to the combination of medications and psychosocial support, such as counseling, but in this book I use it to refer to buprenorphine, methadone, or extended-release naltrexone treatment with or without psychosocial support.

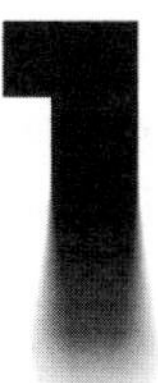

WHAT'S NIXON GOT TO DO WITH IT?

A History of Medication-Assisted Treatment

SHREVEPORT, LOUISIANA, a town founded on an old Caddo Indian settlement on the Red River, had a population of sixteen thousand in 1900. After prospectors discovered crude oil in the area, the Standard Oil Company established a local oil pipeline, causing an employment boom and the city's population to nearly triple during World War I. By 1919, Shreveport supported a symphony orchestra, two colleges, five banks, a state hospital, a federal courthouse, and radio station KWKH, the first in the nation to play phonographic records over the air. Not bad for a city of forty-four thousand people. Through jobs in the oil industry, the population had more money than did neighboring communities.[33]

As was common in America following the Civil War, physicians in Shreveport during the early 1900s widely prescribed morphine to treat a variety of conditions, ranging from pain from a serious injury to menstrual cramps. Shreveport residents tolerated opioid use, even though it was already known to cause addiction. Given frequent morphine prescription for medical ailments, many of Shreveport's residents developed an opioid addiction. These residents came from a variety of professional, economic, and racial backgrounds. Based on records discovered in the 1970s, people with addiction included housewives, politicians, day laborers, waiters, and pretty much every other type of professional common during that time. In an era of zealous Prohibition sentiments, most people with addiction kept their status hidden from their families and friends, with one interesting exception: many revealed their addiction to the family physician.[33]

Few Americans today feel confident having a frank discussion about addiction with their physician, so the patient-physician relationship of the early 1900s may seem surprising. Yet between the Civil War and 1914, physicians routinely prescribed maintenance doses of morphine to people with an addiction to ward off withdrawal symptoms and cravings, allowing people to function in their daily lives. Most maintenance prescribing occurred in private physicians' offices, but some cities, including Jacksonville, Florida, and New York City, had federally funded morphine maintenance clinics. Morphine maintenance was so common that in 1919 the US Supreme Court heard a case on exactly that topic.[33]

In *Webb v. United States*, Dr. Webb, a physician from Shreveport, appealed his conviction of violating the Harrison Narcotics Tax Act of 1914.[34] The Harrison Act, which regulated opioids and other narcotics, was largely a response to anti-immigrant hysteria because Chinese immigrants were stereotyped as smokers of opium. The Harrison Act was one of the first times the federal government regulated the physician-patient relationship. According to the text of the law, a physician could dispense opioids only "during the course of his professional practice." Like many other physicians of his era, Dr. Webb had interpreted the Harrison Act to allow morphine maintenance. After all, it was part of his professional medical practice. Unfortunately for Dr. Webb, the Supreme Court disagreed in a five to four vote. The justices argued that morphine maintenance was not a legitimate medical practice, thereby implying that addiction was not a legitimate medical condition. Therefore, any physician prescribing morphine to a known addict was violating the Harrison Act, resulting in a criminal offense.

In 1922, the Supreme Court went even further, stating that no physician could prescribe opioids for any purpose to people with known opioid addiction; eventually, the latter case would be reversed, but by then the harm was already done. Morphine maintenance all but ceased across the country. According to historian William White, "If one were to inquire why the modern physician is so ambivalent about the addicted patient, one would only have to look at the history of 20th century medicine."[35] It was not until the 1970s that the US federal government re-permitted opioid maintenance, albeit in a highly restricted manner within methadone clinics.

Even before the *Webb* case, agents of the Federal Bureau of Narcotics (FBN), a predecessor to today's Drug Enforcement Administration, preemptively interpreted the Harrison Act as banning morphine maintenance. They were busy arresting physicians, often by using informants with opioid addiction to entrap physicians in exchange for freedom. The FBN justified its actions based on the failures of one poorly run maintenance clinic: the New York City maintenance clinic. With far too high a patient-to-physician ratio, limited patient oversight, and an unreasonably high dosage of morphine prescribed, this clinic became the poster child for the supposed dangers of morphine maintenance.[33]

In Louisiana, despite the Supreme Court's interpretation of the Harrison Act, the state Board of Health voted to allow Shreveport to open a morphine maintenance clinic. The board feared that an arbitrary end to the practice would cause a surge in addiction-related social problems, from unemployment to petty theft. By designating one physician to control prescriptions and by limiting dispensing to one drugstore, the board believed it could exert enough control to placate federal agents.[33]

Dr. Willis P. Butler was chosen to run this clinic. A soft-spoken, strong-willed Louisiana native, Dr. Butler was one of Shreveport's most respected residents. After working as a druggist's assistant, supporting himself through medical school, and serving as a country physician, he began an illustrious career, including serving in political positions for forty-eight years.[33]

Despite the general cultural animosity toward people with addiction, Shreveport's maintenance clinic was widely lauded by the community. Dr. Butler was clearly not a quack, nor was he in it for the money since the clinic primarily provided free treatment supported by state funds. Even the sheriff and local judges believed the clinic decreased drug-related criminal behavior, making their jobs easier. Local physicians likewise appreciated the opportunity to outsource addiction care while continuing to see those same patients for other diseases. Decades later, the nonprofit Drug Abuse Council examined the clinic's medical records and concluded, "These addicts were able to live, work, and lead quite normal and productive lives while being maintained."[33]

By the end of the clinic's first year, 460 Shreveport residents had received maintenance morphine, though this number is probably an underestimate since the clinic did not record transient people. Dr. Butler's clinic also treated venereal diseases, such as syphilis. Importantly, if politics surrounding maintenance were to become dicey, the state would continue paying staff to treat venereal diseases while the staff unofficially managed addiction. The clinic also offered an early form of case management, helping patients find employment, for example.[33]

Local newspapers praised Dr. Butler's clinic. In response to fears that federal agents would shut the clinic down, in 1920 the *Shreveport Journal* published an editorial supporting the clinic's continuation. In the meantime, major reorganization was taking place in the Federal Bureau of Narcotics, with Prohibition zealots redirecting federal drug policy toward an "abstinence only" policy.[33]

Depending on whom you talked to in the bureau, addiction was one of two things: a moral and criminal failing requiring punishment or a disease requiring a cure through detoxification followed by education and recuperation. The FBN saw morphine maintenance as neither punishment nor cure, and thus as ineffective and dangerous. In contrast, Dr. Butler and other physicians firmly believed that addiction was a disease and that some people with addiction would never be "cured." His staff would assess whether patients were "curable" or "incurable." Curable patients, the majority in Shreveport, were sent to detoxification in an associated hospital followed by rehabilitation. Incurable patients were provided with daily maintenance doses of morphine, enough to keep them functional while controlling cravings and withdrawal without causing a high. As might be expected, the FBN had few problems with detoxification but battled the maintenance clinic at every turn. Within a few years, they succeeded in shutting the clinic down, leaving many people with opioid addiction no effective options.[33]

The bureau thought curbing the opioid supply would halt addiction; instead, it merely increased crime. According to David Musto, who served as drug policy advisor to President Jimmy Carter, the closing of early-twentieth-century maintenance clinics like Shreveport's caused opioid prices in the illicit market to immediately spike by as much as 50 percent across the country, contributing to a thriving black market.[36] One would have expected policy makers at the time to take notice, but decades passed until opioid maintenance was seriously discussed at the national level.

FROM THE HARRISON ACT in 1914 through the early 1960s, policy makers viewed opioid addiction almost entirely through a criminal lens with a goal of decreasing the supply of drugs rather than decreasing the demand for drugs. The chief public health villain of the time was Henry Anslinger, a bald-headed master of propaganda and commissioner of the Federal Bureau of Narcotics. Anslinger was responsible for perceptions of "reefer madness," the supposed psychosis resulting from marijuana use. His propaganda resulted in a serious documentary about marijuana, which is now considered a comedy cult classic due to its unsupported horrific claims, including cannabis-induced murderous rages. Anslinger urged Congress to institute mandatory two-year drug sentences for first-time drug offenses and to make heroin sales to minors punishable by death.[35]

Even before maintenance clinics had disappeared, Anslinger viewed them as "supply depots" and "barrooms for addicts."[35] With maintenance clinic closures, people suffering from addiction had few places to turn. Hospitals frequently barred patients considered "immoral," including people with addiction. Jails and prisons were the primary addiction intake facilities of the time, giving temporary reprieve from active drug use while ostracizing people and converting some into hardcore criminals.

By the late 1920s, federal prisons were asking the federal government to segregate people with addiction, who represented most of the incarcerated population. In response, Congress allocated funds to construct two "narcotic farms," federally funded treatment centers for prisoners that also accepted voluntary participants from the public. One narcotic farm was based in Fort Worth, Texas; the other was in Lexington, Kentucky. With barred windows and gates, the Lexington facility clearly resembled a prison, except that it housed a library and research laboratories. Unlike most prisons at the time, it also employed physicians, nurses, social workers, and therapists whose collective goal was to treat addiction. Treatment methods consisted of detoxification and convalescence, as well as vocational activities, such as farming, therapy and support groups, and recreational activities. Since it voluntarily accepted patients, the Lexington facility saw many jazz musicians make their way through too, and it earned a reputation around the country as a mecca of jazz since musicians were encouraged to practice for hours during daily treatment.[37]

Ultimately, 90 percent of the Lexington narcotic farm population relapsed upon release, partly due to no existing follow-up care.[35] Nevertheless, research conducted at these narcotic farms proved instrumental in later advances in addiction treatment.

DR. JEROME H. JAFFE was a stereotypical scientist: pale from spending most of his time in the lab and bespectacled in gold-rimmed glasses. He was logical, analytical, and blunt—exactly the type of person you would want directing drug policy. The son of a Jewish Lithuanian immigrant grocer, he had been urged by his father to become a doctor. Instead, Jaffe wanted to become an auto mechanic but had difficulty finding a job. Rather than argue with his parents, he signed up for some premed courses at Temple University and quickly found an interest in psychology. After earning a master's degree, he realized there were more resources available for people studying medicine than psychology, so he applied for medical school and paid his way through by playing music at weddings.[38] During his last semester of medical school, he did some pharmacology research and found it fascinating.

In the early 1960s, after graduating from medical school and serving a brief internship in a Staten Island hospital, Jaffe was accepted into the clinical division of the addiction treatment center at the Lexington narcotic farm, a wing where patients volunteered to participate in addiction research. As a federal prison, the Lexington narcotic farm fulfilled Jaffe's military obligation to work in public health service. More importantly, it allowed him to be in the same location as one of his idols, Abraham Wikler, a famous scholar of psychiatric medications.[39] Jaffe would later describe the narcotic farm as the "center of the world for learning about drug addiction."

Rather than landing in the research division at the Lexington narcotic farm, however, Jaffe was placed in a clinical position. A pharmacologist at heart, he would have much preferred the research division, but the clinical position gave him an opportunity to see opioid addiction in action, teaching him about concepts such as withdrawal, tolerance, and craving. Fortunately for Jaffe, the clinicians and researchers met regularly during lunch, cross-pollinating ideas about addiction treatment.[39]

To his knowledge, Jaffe had never met anyone with an opioid addiction, but he found that people with the condition were likeable and not that different from the rest of the people he knew. He also saw the brutality of opioid addiction—how difficult it was to simply "quit" once one had become dependent. Searching for a treatment, he became interested in a medication called methadone.

At the time, scientists knew little about opioid receptors in the brain, but they knew that there was something special about methadone,[39] specifically that it prevented withdrawal symptoms and was well-liked by the research subjects.[37] Methadone is an opioid with a long half-life, meaning its effects last a long time as it is slowly eliminated from blood plasma, thus preventing the frequent physiological ups and downs associated with shorter-lasting opioids, such as heroin. Jaffe observed that someone using heroin might seek a new dose every few hours to prevent painful withdrawal symptoms and to keep cravings at bay, but someone taking methadone would feel stable the entire day. Over time Jaffe's faith in methadone as an addiction treatment grew, but he was also convinced that psychological treatment was needed to complement it.[35,38,40]

Jaffe and other scientists were likely able to study methadone's effects, despite the federal ban on opioid maintenance treatment, because methadone formed the crux of a research study at a federally funded institution. However, the studies were not without ethical controversy. Even though prisoners had voluntarily provided consent, some prisoners may have incorrectly believed participation would cut time from their sentences.[38] But according to Jaffe, it was a different era and the federal regulations of ethics in research that exist today did not exist back then.[38] Additionally, a minority of Lexington participants were rewarded for their participation with morphine that they could use to get high on for special occasions and holidays.[41] The Lexington narcotic farm eventually closed in the 1970s, when a national network of treatment centers supplanted it.

Jaffe was not the only one exploring methadone's effects on opioid addiction during the 1960s. In the Upper East Side of Manhattan at Rockefeller University, Vincent P. Dole, a metabolic specialist, and Marie Nyswander, a psychiatrist, were experimenting with methods to stabilize people suffering from opioid addiction. First, the researchers tried regular heroin doses but found that heroin's short half-life resulted in a fast return of withdrawal symptoms and cravings. Moreover, people quickly grew tolerant of heroin, necessitating higher, potentially life-threatening doses. Overall, patients seemed to grow less stable, not more stable. Next, the researchers tried morphine, but the same pattern developed as with heroin. What they needed was an opioid with a long half-life, thereby preventing the ups and downs of withdrawal and cravings, as well as an opioid that produced minimal tolerance.[35,40]

Like Jaffe, Dole and Nyswander studied methadone as a potential option. Because their patients already had so much heroin and morphine in their systems, they required high doses of methadone for stabilization. Yet despite the high dose, patients did not grow tolerant of methadone's effects. Tolerance would have required ever escalating doses. Furthermore, methadone's side effects were minimal. Most importantly, patients stopped having withdrawal symptoms and cravings long enough for them to function during the day. Like Dr. Butler decades before him, Dole believed that these patients with severe addiction had a chronic, incurable disease. Dole called his treatment method "methadone maintenance."[35,40]

Having learned of Dole and Nyswander's experiments, Jaffe's confidence in methadone's potential blossomed. Unlike Dole and Nyswander, however, he did not think that inpatient hospital administration of methadone was necessary. Conducting his own experiment, he wrote methadone prescriptions for his patients on prescription pads in his outpatient office. Patients would get methadone from the local pharmacy and return to his office for medication management, which included dosage adjustments, urine drug screenings, and counseling. This approach allowed Jaffe's patients to live with their families and to participate in the workforce.[42]

In 1968, Jaffe opened a pilot program in Chicago called the Illinois Drug Abuse Program (IDAP), essentially a research laboratory sanctioned by the Illinois legislature.[38] IDAP consisted of three alternative programs: an outpatient methadone maintenance program that clients attended daily, a brief inpatient detoxification program, and a residential therapeutic community. The therapeutic community was modeled on a program called Daytop, which itself was modeled on a notorious program called Synanon.[39]

Synanon was a program formed by people who identified as "ex-addicts." Their leader was Charles Dederich, a man who would at one point attain rock-star status only to fall from public favor as a disgraced "cult" leader. Among other bizarre actions, he armed his therapeutic residential facility, required participants to shave their heads, and mandated sterilization and abortions. Synanon viewed addiction as rooted in immaturity, immorality, and irresponsibility. A rigid lifestyle of privileges and punishments to incentivize proper behavior would supposedly transform the individual into an upstanding citizen. Synanon's best-known feature was adversarial confrontation, in which participants broke each other down and built each other back up by spewing insults until they were forced to be honest with themselves and the group.[43] Unlike Synanon, the therapeutic community in Jaffe's IDAP program kept confrontation to a minimum. Also in contrast to Synanon, Jaffe's therapeutic community permitted the use of methadone treatment.[38] Though a philosophical battle existed at the time between proponents of therapeutic communities and proponents of methadone treatment, Jaffe felt the modalities could be combined and that people who relapsed following one approach could try the other.[38]

A researcher at heart, Jaffe hoped to test the effectiveness of IDAP's three modalities, so he randomly assigned patients to one of the three programs. Of course, patients had their own preferences and sometimes became frustrated with this approach. Nevertheless, IDAP quickly became popular, leading Jaffe to open a second branch serving five hundred people. Eventually even more branches were opened. Knowing that addiction is a chronic, relapsing disease, Jaffe created a special "barebones" unit for patients who had dropped out of the program or had been forced out for behavioral problems but who wanted to try treatment again. A stepping-stone to full participation, the barebones unit acknowledged the relapsing, chronic nature of addiction.[39,42] In some ways, it was a precursor to "low-barrier" medication-assisted treatment programs that exist today.

WHEN ANSLINGER RETIRED IN 1964, attitudes in Washington, DC, relaxed somewhat toward drug users. The Supreme Court ruled that being addicted was not illegal, even though illicit drug possession continued to be a criminal offense. The National Institute of Mental Health, an agency predominantly concerned with health matters and filled with psychologists, took over some of the Federal Bureau of Narcotics' responsibilities. Perhaps most surprisingly, in 1963 a presidential advisory commission recommended a treatment approach rather than a criminal justice approach to the drug problem,[42] forming the seeds of a public health slant to drug policy. In retrospect, President Richard Nixon hardly seemed like the man to plant them.

Having grown up in the Anslinger era, Nixon began his presidency with what Michael Massing calls a "reflexive disgust for illegal drugs and the people who used them."[42] Nixon associated drugs with hippies, a population with whom he felt nothing in common. His presidential campaign rhetoric only described a supply-side approach—increasing the number of border control agents and cooperating internationally to halt the drug trade. Nixon was especially obsessed with destroying the "French connection," a heroin trafficking scheme among Turkey, France, and the United States.

To serve on his domestic policy staff, Nixon chose Jeff Donfeld, who happened to be dating Nixon's daughter. Donfeld was the opposite of a hippie: sober, affluent, and conservative. In some respects, he was a younger version of Nixon. In the White House, Donfeld worked for a former football coach, Bud Wilkinson, to whom Nixon had assigned drug policy development. Wilkinson's plan focused on informing Americans that drugs are bad.

Even though Donfeld felt no empathy for drug users, he thought Wilkinson's scare-tactic educational approach an ineffective solution to a complex problem. So Donfeld began reading research articles about addiction treatment on his own, including articles about methadone. His interest in methadone treatment quickly grew when he read that it was correlated with lower crime and higher employment—two key goals of the Nixon administration.[38,42]

The nation's crime rate had doubled, including in Washington, DC, and Nixon wanted to be the president who curbed crime. Local criminal justice initiatives such as reorganizing DC's courts and hiring additional police officers did not appear to be working, necessitating a new approach.

Nixon tasked his advisor, John Ehrlichman, with finding a solution. Ehrlichman, in turn, looked to his young aide, Egil Krogh, who asked Donfeld for advice. Donfeld described the methadone literature he'd read. Krogh, despite having grown up as a Christian Scientist who abstained from all mind-altering substances, was favorably impressed. To further examine the possibility of methadone as a solution to the crime problem, Krogh contacted Robert DuPont, an addiction treatment expert and psychiatrist who had experience treating addiction with methadone in the DC Department of Corrections.[38,42]

I recently had the privilege of interviewing DuPont, who said to me, "I believe I'm the only person in the world who has known all seventeen White House drug czars." Clearly passionate about improving the lives of drug users, DuPont described in fascinating detail the political dynamics of methadone treatment during the Nixon era, a time when some US scholars were arguing for the adoption of the British system with legalized prescription heroin. DuPont's experience with methadone treatment began in the Department of Corrections, because "I cared about the prisoners and I wanted to help them."

DuPont invited Krogh to visit the Department of Corrections and to speak with patients on methadone treatment; Krogh listened sympathetically to their experiences. Impressed with DuPont's program, Krogh helped DuPont obtain funding to open the first DC methadone clinic outside of the criminal justice system. With an air of amusement during our interview, DuPont remarked, "People say Corrections are bad guys! Hey, Corrections is where it started!"

In part, DuPont had garnered Krogh's attention by emphasizing the link between heroin addiction and crime. In retrospect, the link between heroin addiction and crime seems obvious, but prior to Nixon the federal government tended to see both issues separately. For over a decade, DuPont had desired to develop innovative treatment programs with methadone in the Department of Corrections, but under Lyndon B. Johnson no one was interested. Johnson's DC Crime Commission report barely even mentioned drugs.

But Nixon's administration moved the issue of crime to the center of politics. Convinced that treatment was a way to address crime, the Nixon administration enabled DuPont to have the funding he wanted by 1969. Furthermore, Nixon's White House worked with people from across the political spectrum to address crime. DuPont said, "I was thirty-seven, and they noticed me. I'm a Democrat, but they didn't care about what party I was in. I didn't care what party they were in. I was on a mission and they were on a mission." Describing Krogh, DuPont says, "He was a wonderful guy and had a terrible outcome in his life because he was involved with the plumbers and all that stuff," referring to Krogh's later imprisonment for his part in the Watergate scandal.

DuPont obtained federal funding for a citywide methadone program, which almost instantly reached two thousand patients. Even though the White House, the DC mayor, and the DC chief of police all supported DuPont's methadone program, others in the city did not. DuPont became the focus of significant negative publicity and even death threats.

One day in the early 1970s, George Allen, a reporter from a widely watched DC television station, asked DuPont for an in-person interview. During the interview, DuPont explained the methadone program's benefits, including an already evident decrease in crime rates and overdose rates. Allen looked DuPont in the eye and said, "You're a liar." Shortly thereafter, Allen's television station aired a prime-time documentary about the DC methadone clinic, in which DuPont and his program were described as a fraud.

Interestingly, Katharine Graham, the woman who owned the *Washington Post* and oversaw publication of the Watergate scandal, also owned Allen's television station. Following the negative prime-time documentary, editors at the *Washington Post* contacted Graham, explaining that Allen was wrong and DuPont was right. The editors asked for permission to correct the record by writing a piece in the *Post*. Graham gave them permission to criticize the television station she owned, saying, "Do what you need to do." According to DuPont, the *Washington Post* piece squashed Allen's reputation: "Boom, end of the issue. It was extremely dramatic. He left town. He was gone."

Unfortunately, the focus on methadone as a social tool rather than as a method of improving the quality of individual drug users' lives lent the medication racist overtones. Many African American inner-city residents viewed methadone skeptically or with outright animosity, with prominent community leaders and the Black Panther Party claiming that methadone was an attempt by whites to control blacks.[38] The Black Panthers called methadone "chemical warfare" against African Americans.[44] The Congressional Black Caucus argued that substantial federal funds should be used to study the long-term effects of methadone, especially since methadone treatment was primarily available in inner-city, urban areas populated by minorities.[44] Distrust of federally funded treatment programs was also due to revelations of the profound mistreatment of African American males during the Tuskegee Syphilis Study, reports of forced sterilizations, and limited government interest in sickle cell anemia.[44] The Black Panther Party argued that traditional Chinese medicine, such as acupuncture, was a better alternative to methadone treatment, despite lack of evidence of efficacy. Additionally, prominent members of the black community felt that an individualized, medicalized response to addiction ignored racial and social inequalities that contributed to the condition. When I spoke with DuPont, he described an on-air radio interview he once had with Howard University, when a young activist phoned into the station and publicly called for DuPont's death for what the methadone program was doing to the "young negro men of our city." Once it became clear that methadone was here to stay, responses from the African American community ranged from tepid acceptance of the treatment to creation of African American–led methadone treatment centers to replacement of existing programs with alternative methods.[44]

The Nixon administration's financial and political support for methadone treatment in DC represented a seismic shift in federal drug policy. For the first time, addiction treatment would be as important as stopping the illicit drug trade. Furthermore, for the first time since the Harrison Act of 1914, the federal government would fund maintenance clinics, albeit with a far more effective medication for treating addiction.

As expected, DC's methadone clinic had a favorable effect on local crime rates. Regular methadone treatment participants were arrested less frequently than those who dropped out of the program or did not receive methadone at all. Given methadone's local success, Krogh convinced his boss, Ehrlichman, to start a task force to discuss the feasibility of starting methadone treatment programs across the nation. Since participating agencies, such as the National Institute of Mental Health, had never expressed much interest in addiction treatment, Krogh was concerned that they would overlook methadone's potential. So, he set up a parallel secret task force. This second task force, headed by Jaffe, was composed of health experts rather than government workers.[39,42]

The official government task force proposed traditional psychotherapy as the national solution to opioid addiction, reflecting the

National Institute of Mental Health's vested interests and expertise in psychotherapy. The report also expressed doubt in methadone as a treatment for addiction. In contrast, Jaffe's task force believed that opioid addiction is usually resistant to psychotherapy alone, necessitating the addition of medication to control physiological symptoms. Jaffe's task force also extolled methadone's potential to stabilize "hardcore drug addicts," turning them into law-abiding citizens.[39,42] Years later, Jaffe summarized the report as saying "there are an awful lot of people waiting for treatment with methadone and you can't just keep pretending that methadone is a small research project."[38] Additionally, Jaffe's task force argued that the drug problem must be met through a coordinated and integrated national approach that addressed both treatment and prevention.[38]

Based on the two task forces' reports, Donfeld drafted a list of policy options for Nixon's chief domestic advisors. Donfeld praised methadone treatment as an economical and effective crime reduction method. He also proposed a $60 million increase in treatment funding, with a large share dedicated to expanding methadone treatment across the nation. But Nixon's influential Secretary of Health, Education, and Welfare opposed methadone, proposing psychotherapy and therapeutic community approaches instead. Donfeld's argument might have fallen on deaf ears but for a 1971 Congressional investigation into the Vietnam War. The investigation claimed that 10–15 percent of returning Vietnam veterans had heroin addiction. In response, the *New York Times* published "G.I. Heroin Addiction Epidemic in Vietnam" on its front page.[45] There was even talk in Congress of civilly committing returning soldiers.[46]

Although often idealistic, Nixon was a pragmatist at heart. The Vietnam War was already unpopular; knowledge of widespread addiction among vets was threatening to push the public over the edge. Thus, Nixon was open to new ideas, especially cost-effective ones. As the methadone clinic in DC had demonstrated, one methadone clinic could treat two thousand people at a time on an outpatient basis. The other main option under discussion, therapeutic communities, required several months of residential treatment for only a few dozen participants per facility. Nixon gave his blessing to a national methadone treatment program and chose Jaffe, a Democrat, to head it. As a result, between 1970 and 1973, the number of people treated for opioid addiction increased eight-fold nationally.[40] Nixon also chose Jaffe to lead a new office for coordinating drug policy, the Special Action Office for Drug Abuse Prevention, taking the drug issue out of the National Institute of Mental Health's firm grip.[42]

In 1971, Nixon called drug abuse "public enemy number one," necessitating "a new, all-out offensive." This was the beginning of the war on drugs. For his war, Nixon requested $155 million, of which a whopping two-thirds ($105 million) would be earmarked for treatment. By 1973, the federal government would spend $420 million on treatment and prevention alone, an eight-fold increase from when Nixon took office.[42] To this day, no US president since Nixon has ever requested such a large share of the drug policy budget for treatment. In an interview with PBS in 2000 about the Nixon administration, Jaffe reflected:

> I had the feeling, almost from the first day, that the willingness to look at the demand side, rather than the traditional American law enforcement approach might be a transient phenomenon—that it might pass, and we would go back to our old ways of more and more law enforcement. And I was right. We have never had that proportion of federal resources devoted to intervention on the demand side. We'd never had it before, and we've never had it since.[46]

As head of the new government agency in a position referred to as the "drug czar," Jaffe prioritized increasing the number of treatment slots and decreasing wait lists. Funding was allocated to methadone clinics in high-need cities. But clinics had to meet certain conditions, such as retention quotas. If too many patients quit, the government agency would send an investigative team and demand corrective action.[42]

In 1972, the agency passed regulations intended to prevent methadone diversion and ensure an adequate standard of care. Regulations detailed the minimum dosage, defined take-home conditions, and created a closed system wherein methadone could only be dispensed for addiction treatment in special methadone clinics, today called opioid treatment programs, and hospitals. These restrictions are still largely in place, though now through an accreditation system.[47] And methadone for addiction treatment continues to be the most heavily restricted FDA-approved medication.

A firm believer that multiple treatment modalities should be offered and that a "one size fits all" approach is ineffective, Jaffe also expanded the growth of abstinence-only treatment programs, including therapeutic communities. He hated being associated with methadone only.[42]

Public backlash against methadone began quickly, and it's a backlash that continues today. The most pressing concern was diversion to the black market. Jaffe believed the diversion issue was being blown out of proportion, especially given the positive impact methadone had on people with addiction. Adding to Jaffe's stress, infighting was occurring at his government agency, with different people having different agendas and philosophies about drug treatment. The National Institute of Mental Health, for example, routinely refused to cooperate with Jaffe's agency, delaying important treatment contracts. Even though Jaffe's agency was making significant progress toward treatment expansion with wait times across the country decreasing and some treatment centers having excess capacity, methadone's public image was negative overall.[42]

The federal government also continued traditional supply-side approaches of raiding and arresting drug traffickers internationally. The domestic heroin supply declined after government raids destroyed sources in several countries. The combination of treatment expansion and government raids appeared to be reducing crime rates. In 1972, the FBI released a report indicating that crime rates had fallen in 94 of the 154 cities studied, with the largest decline in Washington, DC. Since treatment had received the largest bolster in funding and personnel, it appeared that treatment, rather than government raids, was the true cause of the crime reduction. Even the DC chief of police agreed.[42]

Despite the visible successes of treatment policy, many politicians still favored a punitive approach. In New York, Governor Nelson Rockefeller proposed draconian mandatory sentences for drug-related crimes, including life sentences for possession. Jaffe met with Rockefeller to persuade him of the folly of punitive measures,[39] but Rockefeller rejected Jaffe's arguments, naively believing that mandatory prison sentences would encourage drug users to seek treatment. Of course, Jaffe knew that addiction did not work like this. Nixon also created the Drug Enforcement Administration (DEA) in the Department of Justice whose focus on supply-side initiatives continues today.[39] And Nixon signed the Controlled Substances Act, creating a tier of restrictions for controlled substances depending on their abusability and medical value. The newly created DEA and the already established Food and Drug Administration would jointly decide the position of each drug on the controlled substance schedule. Infamously, marijuana was placed in a more restrictive schedule than some opioids.

By 1973, Jaffe felt overwhelmed with enemies. The public was increasingly antimethadone. Seeing lines of lower-income, sometimes-rowdy people in impoverished neighborhoods, the public associated methadone with crime and immoral behavior, which was ironic given that lower crime rates were attributed to methadone treatment expansion. Nonetheless, city zoning boards were denying the construction of new methadone clinics—something that still happens today.

In addition to public backlash, a clash of philosophies among federal agencies caused incessant infighting, especially between Jaffe's agency and the National Institute of Mental Health. Moreover, Nixon was seriously considering Rockefeller's mandatory minimum sentencing approach, with which Jaffe strongly disagreed. Jaffe's negative opinion of mandatory sentences leaked to the press and was taken as a sign of disloyalty by the Nixon administration.[39] Despite his agency's clear successes, Jaffe sent Nixon a letter of resignation, wishing to return to his first love—research. Unfortunately, Jaffe's departure marked the beginning of a precipitous decline in federal treatment funding and initiatives for addiction treatment.[39]

Under Presidents Gerald Ford and Jimmy Carter, addiction treatment funding in real terms dropped. In response, methadone clinics were closing their doors, including Jaffe's beloved IDAP in Chicago. By 1975, attention previously paid to opioid addiction turned toward marijuana, a drug that public health experts had historically viewed as relatively benign. But parents of teenagers increasingly feared marijuana, and the "parents' movement," bolstered by corporate and religious donations, soon dominated federal drug policy.[42,48]

Nancy Reagan acted as drug policy ambassador under President Ronald Reagan with her infamous "Just Say No" movement. The administration and the message presumed that Americans simply needed drug education and willpower to prevent drug use or overcome addiction. Treatment funding policies reflected Reagan's small government ideal—lower taxes and lower public spending. Why should the government fund treatment, especially for people who disrespect the law? Furthermore, according to the Reagan administration, twelve-step groups were free and had a spiritual approach, prompting participants to reflect on their wrongs and ask for forgiveness, a perfect approach for an administration trying to increase the morality of the nation. On a talk show in Illinois, Nancy Reagan stated, "Alcoholics Anonymous is extremely successful and it's not federally financed. I never thought that money is the answer."[42]

If the First Lady approved of any "professional" treatment, it was boot camps. She supported Straight Inc., which offered "tough love" in an enclosed, prisonlike residential environment. Proud of Straight Inc.'s approach, Nancy took Princess Diana to visit the facility. Resembling Synanon in certain respects, Straight Inc.'s methodology included public confessions, sleep deprivation, education, and constant surveillance. Parents at their wits' ends committed their teens, expecting character transformation and sobriety. In addition to being ineffective, Straight Inc. and similar facilities were highly inequitable, only affordable to upper-class people at the cost of thousands of dollars per month. Like Synanon, they rejected methadone as "just another drug."[42,49]

By 1986, the federal treatment budget in real terms was one-fifth the amount Jaffe had to work with in 1973.[42] The remaining methadone clinics were characterized by long wait lists, high counselor-to-patient ratios, and crumbling buildings. Deprived of funding for ancillary programming, they offered insufficient counseling and case management. These limited services further tarnished the public image of methadone clinics, making them seem like gas stations rather than treatment centers. Even when the HIV/AIDS crisis emerged, the Reagan administration rejected methadone treatment expansion and syringe exchanges for ideological reasons. Both tools would have reduced the spread of HIV/AIDS, saving countless lives.[50]

That same year, the federal government instituted mandatory minimum sentences for drug offenses under the Anti-Drug Abuse Act, further dismantling the public health approach favored by Jaffe. The legislation's cocaine-crack disparity is perhaps its most infamous element. Legislators knew that whites were more likely to use cocaine, and African Americans were more likely to use crack, a cheaper derivative of cocaine. Congress set the per gram prison sentence length for crack at one hundred times the prison sentence for cocaine, disproportionately affecting African Americans.[48] The largest suffering was arguably borne by African American children, whose parents were being incarcerated at ever increasing rates, forcing children into a severely underfunded foster care system.

In 1988, Reagan replaced the agency Jaffe used to run, the Special Action Office for Drug Abuse Prevention, with the Office of National Drug Control Policy. Decades later, under the Obama administration, the Office of National Drug Control Policy would advocate for MAT. Under Reagan, however, the office was led by William Bennett, a man likened to cowboy Clint Eastwood in the film *The Good, the Bad, and the Ugly*, seeing only "good guys" and "bad guys" in the war on drugs. The bad guys included not only drug traffickers and dealers but also drug users and those who looked the other way.[51] Moreover, Bennett viewed drug use as highly contagious, a position for which he had no scientific evidence but that presupposed the need to lock drug users away from society. He considered treatment to be the "coddling" of people who should be taught personal responsibility. Instead, he pushed for an increase in criminal justice initiatives. Like Rockefeller, he explained that even *if* treatment were effective, criminal justice measures would prompt people to quit drugs and enter treatment. Bennett firmly believed that people with addiction would not seek treatment voluntarily.

Therefore, in his 1989 report to the White House, now under George H. W. Bush, Bennett took pains to explain that empowering law enforcement to punish drug dealers and users was actually a demand-side tactic rather than a supply-side tactic. He also argued that shifting funds from law enforcement to treatment would be naïve since treatment programs were already overburdened—obscuring the fact that funding would lead to more treatment slots and staff, thereby enabling treatment programs to become *less* burdened.[52] Ultimately, Bennett proposed spending three-quarters of the federal drug budget on supply-side initiatives and only one-quarter on demand-side initiatives. A small part of the demand-side initiative would be treatment.

Revealingly, when opioid overdoses hit headlines in 2015, Bennett penned an article called "Bring Back the War on Drugs." In it he offered the following advice:

> The heroin epidemic is inflicted upon us by criminal acts that produce an abundant supply of inexpensive drugs. Stopping these criminal acts will stop the epidemic. The Obama administration refuses to do this, insisting that overdose medication and treatment for heroin users and addicts are sufficient. Medication to revive dying addicts will not prevent the explosion of new heroin users, nor will it get addicts truly clean and sober. Emergency triage doesn't immobilize the plague or prevent its spread.[53]

Bennett goes on to say that families with addicted loved ones know the disease is hopeless. He suggests no policies to help Americans already affected by addiction, preferring to protect the uninitiated innocents instead.[53]

When President Bill Clinton took office, two hundred thousand Americans were lingering on drug treatment waiting lists. More inclined toward treatment policies than Reagan or Bush, Clinton proposed a treatment budget increase, primarily by means of state grants. But Congress believed the administration should focus on drug education instead. Politicians shied away from treatment rhetoric, afraid of being perceived as "soft on crime." At most they would support treatment in prison. Ultimately, Congress barely raised funding for treatment, with almost none earmarked to treat people with severe addictions. Democrats were losing their stamina fighting for a demand-side approach. Besides, the public appeared more concerned with marijuana. So Rahm Emanuel, the deputy director of the White House communications office, asked the Office of National Drug Control Policy to focus on marijuana instead.[48]

AS EARLY AS THE 1950s, when methadone's potential was emerging in laboratory and clinical experiments, some governmental research organizations were apprehensive about its safety. Heroin, too, had originally been touted as a safe pharmaceutical, and now it was a national scourge. Organizations ranging from the American Bar Association to the American Medical Association to the National Research Council's Committee on Drug Addiction debated the pros and cons of methadone. Dole and Nyswander, the two scientists who had extensively studied methadone treatment and argued for its expansion, viewed these debates as tainted by political concerns that should have no role in scientific discussions. When the Federal Bureau of Narcotics, which had always been vehemently against opioid maintenance treatment, was eventually replaced by the Drug Enforcement Administration, the DEA adopted its predecessor's distrust of methadone.[54,55]

Given methadone's precarious political and social positions, and despite the Nixon administration's support for methadone, governmental research organizations began an intensive search for alternative addiction treatment medications in the 1970s. They largely focused on antagonists, a class of medications that do not activate opioid receptors in the brain. Antagonists block the brain's opioid receptors, thus preventing a high. One promising candidate was naltrexone.[55] Even though one could technically overdose by using large amounts of opioids while on naltrexone, such a situation was very unlikely given that naltrexone would block an opioid high, thus rendering any opioid use pointless.

The FDA approved naltrexone for opioid addiction treatment in 1984 under the brand name ReVia. But ReVia never really took off among patients or physicians. The problem was you had to take it at home daily, and unlike methadone, it did little for opioid cravings and did not prevent withdrawals. So taking ReVia demanded a tremendous amount of motivation knowing it would block a high without the other benefits of methadone.[55]

Decades later, the FDA approved a long-lasting injectable version of naltrexone under the brand name Vivitrol. Unlike ReVia, which lasts for only twenty-four hours, Vivitrol lasts for twenty-eight days—leading some health providers to tell their patients: "Make one good decision per month, take Vivitrol." Vivitrol is commercially more successful than ReVia, both because patients can better adhere to the medication regimen and because pharmaceutical representatives have targeted criminal justice institutions.[56] Drug courts, prisons, and jails have traditionally opposed methadone and buprenorphine treatment for ideological and practical reasons, but they increasingly view Vivitrol as an appropriate medication for addiction treatment—its main selling point being that it is not an opioid.[56] However, as a more recent medication, extended-release naltrexone has a smaller evidence base than methadone or buprenorphine-naloxone.[57] Few studies have directly compared the efficacy of extended-release naltrexone to other forms of MAT, but existing studies suggest similar efficacy to daily buprenorphine-naloxone for patients.[58,59] Still, extended-release naltrexone appears to have a higher dropout rate after treatment initiation, and dropout may lead to relapse and overdose.[58,60] Additionally, a recent study found that during medication utilization, buprenorphine was more protective against opioid overdose than extended-release naltrexone.[60] Therefore, it seems that activating the opioid receptors in addiction treatment is important for many patients.

RESEARCHERS AND THE National Institute on Drug Abuse were considering the possibility of buprenorphine for addiction treatment during the 1980s and the 1990s. Like methadone, buprenorphine is an opioid, meaning it activates the opioid receptors in the brain, keeping cravings and withdrawal symptoms at bay. Unlike methadone it has a "ceiling effect," meaning that after a certain dosage its effect plateaus, so people have little reason to take too much. As a result, buprenorphine is far less likely than other opioids to lead to respiratory depression, making it one of the safest opioids with a far lower overdose risk than others.[61,62] Furthermore, buprenorphine has greater affinity for the brain's opioid receptors than other opioids, meaning it binds more tightly to the receptors, so it displaces other opioids already on the brain's receptors, after which it blocks the effects of subsequent opioids.[62] Finally, even though buprenorphine has greater *affinity* for the opioid receptor, it actually has weaker intrinsic *activity* at the opioid receptors relative to methadone, meaning it creates less cellular activity, so people with opioid use disorder (OUD) taking buprenorphine as prescribed are less likely to feel euphoria than people taking methadone as prescribed.[12]

Buprenorphine had previously been approved in the United States and France as a pain management medication, albeit at a different dosage and frequency than for addiction treatment. For years in France, it had been prescribed off-label, meaning doctors were prescribing it for addiction treatment without approval. The HIV/AIDS crisis, associated with syringe sharing, eventually propelled France toward prioritizing opioid addiction treatment, resulting in France being the first country to formally approve buprenorphine for that purpose in the 1990s. Buprenorphine's approval and widespread availability was associated with an 80 percent decrease in French deaths from heroin overdose.[63,64] These statistics were hard for American politicians and researchers to ignore.

American researchers and regulators were carefully watching the French story unfold. But to meet the stringent US regulatory requirements, more studies of buprenorphine's efficacy and safety were needed. So, for one of the first times in US history, an American government agency, the National Institute on Drug Abuse, collaborated with a pharmaceutical company, Reckitt & Colman, to test and bring a pharmaceutical to market.[55] In 2002, the FDA approved buprenorphine for addiction treatment, marking the first approval of an opioid for this purpose since methadone in 1972. It was approved under two brand names: Suboxone, which also contained the abuse-deterrent ingredient naloxone, and Subutex, which lacked naloxone but was more appropriate for some populations, such as pregnant women.

In my interview with DuPont, I asked him whether the FDA approval of buprenorphine was as politically contentious as the expansion of methadone into addiction treatment. He responded, "Buprenorphine never had anything like the methadone problem. It was never particularly controversial. You didn't have people saying that you got to kill this guy because he's treating people with buprenorphine. That never happened. But buprenorphine is a really interesting story because it's so different from methadone. Methadone is a program, and buprenorphine is a prescription. That's a big deal."

Anticipating buprenorphine's FDA approval, the DEA, which continued to be unsupportive of maintenance treatment, rescheduled buprenorphine from Schedule V to Schedule III on the federal list of controlled substances. This made the medication more heavily regulated since Schedule III is more restrictive than Schedule V. Even though addiction treatment does require a higher dosage of buprenorphine than is required for pain treatment, DEA transcripts reveal that the rescheduling decision was primarily based on the target population—people with addiction versus people with pain. Unfortunately, people with addiction are significantly less sympathy-endearing. Despite overwhelming objection from the medical community, the DEA wrote, "Simply stated, providing an abusable substance to known drug abusers imparts enhanced risks [sic]."[65] Not for the first time, treatment for a substance use disorder would be regulated more heavily than treatments for other chronic medical conditions. The regulatory outcome could have been even worse. In an interview with *STAT News*, a former director of the National Institute on Drug Abuse said it took substantial advocacy to prevent the DEA from classifying buprenorphine as a Schedule II drug.[66]

Additionally, the DEA worried that the opioid naïve, meaning those not already addicted to opioids, would access buprenorphine to get high. The DEA acted on this concern despite explicitly acknowledging that "the extent to which buprenorphine is able to produce euphoria and 'good drug' effects limits its use by opioid tolerant abusers."[55,65,67] Like Bennett, the DEA prioritized the lives of the uninitiated innocents over those who had already developed a chronic, deadly disease.

Also anticipating buprenorphine's FDA approval, Congress began to rethink existing addiction treatment regulations. The core of the Harrison Act of 1914 was still in effect, prohibiting physicians from prescribing opioids for maintenance treatment in their offices. Methadone, for example, could only be prescribed for addiction treatment in highly regulated methadone clinics to which participants returned daily and waited in visible, stigmatizing lines. Appearing to be outside of mainstream medicine, such clinics attracted few prescribers.

Therefore, starting in the 1990s, buprenorphine's manufacturer urged Congressional staff to amend existing law, an effort that took nearly half a decade.[47] Finally in 2000, Congress passed the Drug Addiction Treatment Act (DATA). It had two goals: to increase opioid maintenance treatment availability and to prevent diversion or abuse. On balance, Congress erred too far on the side of caution, preventing buprenorphine treatment from becoming mainstream medical practice despite proof of its efficacy in increasing health outcomes and preventing overdose.[67]

To prevent diversion of the medication, Congress required any physician prescribing buprenorphine for addiction to obtain a waiver (sometimes called a SAMHSA waiver, after the agency that grants it, or a DATA waiver, after the statute). To obtain this waiver, physicians need special education beyond a standard medical license, typically an additional eight-hour course. Furthermore, and most atypically, in the same statute, Congress instituted patient limits, prohibiting physician practices from prescribing buprenorphine for addiction to more than thirty patients at any time. These patient limits and the education requirements did not apply to prescriptions of buprenorphine for pain management.

The thirty-patient limit applied to entire physician practices rather than to individual physicians. Therefore, if a group of three physicians shared a practice and one had already reached the thirty-patient limit, then the other physicians could not prescribe buprenorphine. Almost immediately, addiction treatment advocates and professional health organizations, including the American Medical Association and the American Society of Addiction Medicine, fought back. They called the restriction arbitrary (why thirty patients?) and dangerous, as it would prevent lifesaving treatment for countless patients. Buprenorphine was, and still is, the only medication in the United States with federal patient limits. Patient limits do not even apply to oxycodone, a medication in Schedule II, a more restrictive schedule than buprenorphine's Schedule III. And oxycodone is often the medication that people undergoing buprenorphine treatment are trying to quit.[67,*]

Given the uproar of public health advocates, Congress amended the rules somewhat in 2005, making the thirty-patient limit apply to individual physicians rather than to entire physician practices.[68] In 2006, after renewed pressure from public health advocates and professional organizations, Congress changed the rules again. This time, individual physicians could prescribe buprenorphine to thirty patients at a time during their first year of having a DATA waiver, and beginning in year two, they could request an expansion, prescribing up to one hundred patients at a time.[69] Senator Orrin Hatch praised the amendment to DATA, saying, "It is clear this [thirty-patient] cap

---

* It is exactly this legal anomaly that prompted my initial foray into public health research, leading to my dissertation and eventually this book. As a trained attorney, I had difficulty understanding how a Schedule III medication was harder to access than a deadlier and more addictive Schedule II medication. Only one factor seemed to explain the anomaly: stigmatization of the patient population.

needs to be raised. To make an analogy, a doctor would not turn away a broken arm because he or she had already fixed thirty arms that month! The doctor would not stand for it, and neither would society. The same should be true for physicians treating drug addiction. Given that the destructive effects of drug addiction are so much greater than a broken arm, we should strive to ensure that the healing hands of doctors are not bound by unintended mandates."[70]

But even with the new rule, wait lists for buprenorphine treatment formed across the country.[71] And wait lists could last a long time. Addiction, after all, is a chronic condition, so a patient can occupy a prescribing slot for years. Unsurprisingly, limited legal access to buprenorphine contributed to buprenorphine prescription sharing, a form of illicit diversion, between family members and friends. Reports emerged of family members and friends forced to negotiate who would take the only available slot, sometimes with tragic consequences. Many people began purchasing buprenorphine illicitly on the street, often to begin recovery or to prevent "dope sickness" or withdrawal symptoms when they could not access buprenorphine legally. Those who sold buprenorphine on the street frequently did so to make money to buy substances, such as heroin, to get high. Others sold parts of prescriptions to afford doctor visits, especially if their doctors did not take insurance, an unethical practice among many buprenorphine prescribers who likely knew they were forcing patients into the black market.[61,72–74]

Illicit diversion has had terrible consequences for the treatment's reputation, perpetuating the myth that buprenorphine is "just another drug." According to an argument I have frequently heard from criminal justice employees, buprenorphine is sold by drug dealers on the street, so it must be the same. In response to diversion concerns, some state legislatures have proposed drastic laws to further restrict buprenorphine treatment. For example, the Indiana legislature recently considered a bill limiting buprenorphine to people addicted for more than one year and over the age of eighteen,[75] despite evidence of efficacy in younger populations.[76,77] The bill would also create a state registry of buprenorphine patients—something that would inevitably decrease the number of patients seeking treatment. Methadone is underused in part because people with previous criminal justice system involvement fear being on a government "watch list." Previous proposed bills in Indiana also attempted to encourage physicians to prescribe extended-release naltrexone (i.e., Vivitrol), which the bills called a "non-addictive" medication, rather than buprenorphine.[78] Enraged, one Indiana addiction psychiatrist told me during an interview, "Politicians should stop dictating my job!"

By 2016, the media was widely reporting on the opioid crisis, focusing on overdoses among upper- and middle-class white Americans. In response, the federal government was taking the opioid crisis seriously. The Obama administration had selected Michael Botticelli as its "drug czar," the position originally held by Jaffe. Botticelli had a history of alcohol addiction that in his early life had resulted in an arrest for driving under the influence. In recovery himself, Botticelli prioritized MAT expansion, calling it "our best hope of making a difference [in overdose deaths]."[79,80] In the Obama administration Nora Volkow continued to head the National Institute on Drug Addiction. A world-renowned physician (and great-granddaughter of Russian socialist revolutionary Leon Trotsky), she has repeatedly called opioid addiction a "brain disease" that can be effectively treated with medications.[81]

In this climate of public health initiatives, politicians began to shed their fear of appearing soft on crime by openly demanding treatment expansion. Emboldened, governors from some of the hardest hit states, such as Vermont, initiated novel programs to expand MAT access.[82] Unlike the Nixon administration, the Obama administration, at least in its rhetoric, prioritized drug users' health over the effect of drugs on crime or unemployment. Recovery of the drug-using individual seemed to be as important as community prosperity.

In 2016, President Barack Obama signed the Comprehensive Addiction and Recovery Act, which for the first time significantly reformed buprenorphine regulations. The act permitted nurse practitioners and physician assistants to prescribe buprenorphine for addiction treatment, subject to any additional rules imposed by the states. For more than a decade, the previous federal law, DATA, had barred physician assistants and nurse practitioners from prescribing buprenorphine, even when states allowed them to prescribe oxycodone. Today, there are still too few nurse practitioners and physician assistants treating addiction, but the Comprehensive Addiction and Recovery Act represents a significant opportunity to expand the addiction treatment workforce.[83]

The new law also permitted a very small percentage of physicians, basically those with board-certified addiction treatment specialization, to treat up to 275 people at any time with buprenorphine.[83] Though a step forward, the law continues buprenorphine's status as the only medication to which patient limits apply. The topic of loosening buprenorphine's regulations is now once again picking up speed. In 2019, top health officials in eighteen states, three US territories, and the District of Columbia wrote to health secretary Alex Azar urging him to relax restrictions. In the letter, the undersigned argue the following:

> The DATA 2000 regulatory framework was implemented prior to the current wave of opioid addiction. The limitations in the legislation and regulations have been intended to preserve safety and to promote comprehensive care. The need for buprenorphine has grown exponentially, while the supply of waived prescribers' pales in comparison. . . . Ideally, legislation should be passed eliminating the waiver requirements and allowing all practitioners who are registered with the Drug Enforcement Administration (DEA) to prescribe controlled substances to also prescribe buprenorphine for the treatment of OUD.

> Researchers in policy have noted that the waiver requirements are burdensome and reduce prescribing. They have also suggested that deregulating buprenorphine would help in reducing stigma associated with treating OUD.[84]

In 2016, Obama signed the 21st Century Cures Act into law, promising $1 billion to state addiction treatment and prevention initiatives.[85] In his 2016 proposed budget, Obama allocated more drug policy dollars toward demand-side initiatives than any other president since Nixon, even though Nixon's percentage allocation toward treatment was still greater.[86,87]

Thus far, President Donald Trump has done far less to address opioid addiction, though he has only been in office for a few years. Trump's commission on the opioid crisis did suggest MAT expansion—a good sign.[88] Likewise, Trump's FDA commissioner, Scott Gottlieb, has openly encouraged MAT expansion and development of new addiction treatment medications.[26] But given existing restrictions on methadone and buprenorphine, pharmaceutical companies are unlikely to view addiction treatment as profitable.[47] Moreover, Trump has declared opioid addiction a national health emergency without the funding to address the emergency. Trump's most positive impact on the opioid crisis so far has been signing into law the SUPPORT for Patients and Communities Act in October 2018. The law included important changes to previous Medicaid restrictions on the number of funded beds in residential treatment centers but did not substantially increase funding to address the crisis. Keith Humphreys, a well-regarded health services researcher who worked on passing the law, said it had "many small sanities" but reflected the ongoing disagreements between Democrats, who traditionally want greater government involvement in addressing public health crises, and Republicans, who traditionally want less.[89] Basically, the parties found agreement on "second tier issues." Most alarmingly, the Trump administration continues its efforts to dismantle the Affordable Care

Act, including by quashing Medicaid expansion. Yet without health insurance, evidence-based addiction treatment is an elusive fantasy for millions of Americans.[90]

ACCESS TO ADDICTION TREATMENT today is far less rosy than the above policy trajectory may imply. Decades of research studies have clarified MAT's lifesaving potential beyond any reasonable doubt. Yet methadone remains inaccessible to most Americans. Many states have only a handful of methadone clinics and one state, Wyoming, has none.[91] When available, methadone clinics often resemble Soviet breadlines—a result of stringent legal regulations separating methadone treatment from office-based practices and requiring daily visits, coupled with clinics only staying open for a few hours each day. Methadone clinics are widely criticized for providing inadequate behavioral health and case management services, often due to inadequate funding.[47] This combination of lines and limited service further cements the public perception of methadone clinics as ineffective fueling stations. Yet unbeknownst to much of the public, methadone has the strongest evidence base of any opioid addiction treatment.[13,22,92]

Buprenorphine, despite the attention afforded it by the Obama administration, is still only prescribed by a minuscule percentage of practicing physicians: approximately 2 percent.[93] It is typically only available in white, middle-class, and upper-class residential areas[93] and rarely in rural areas.[93–96] Even though extended-release naltrexone has no patient limits or special prescribing requirements, only 1 percent of Americans in opioid addiction treatment receive it.[97] And most damning of all, only 20 percent of Americans with opioid addiction receive any treatment whatsoever.[98]

Failed drug policies are often the result of misguided goals. For decades, the federal government focused on decreasing the total number of Americans who start illicit drug use, particularly casual marijuana users who represented the majority of illicit drug users.

Policies included wasting billions of taxpayer dollars on ineffective educational programs about the dangers of drugs,[99] incarcerating people for minor drug offenses, and targeting foreign drug sources with military action. Of course, evidence-based prevention policies should be implemented, but historically US prevention policies have been more motivated by political grandstanding and emotion than by science. Furthermore, the focus on criminal justice supply-side initiatives has stigmatized addiction, preventing treatment-seeking behavior by people with addiction, treatment provision by providers, and treatment funding by policy makers.

In contrast, a goal of managing chronic, severe drug addiction would have necessitated a far different set of policies. People addicted to opioids are typically aware of the drug's dangers. They have frequently already lost their jobs, broken their families, or been involved in the criminal justice system. They continue to use opioids because addiction, by definition, is a disease of compulsive use despite negative consequences, not because they are unaware of the negative consequences or because they are bad people. Educating people with an addiction about the dangers of drugs or putting them in jail are therefore largely ineffective. Likewise, simply restricting the supply of one opioid often leads to substitution with other opioids or other drugs—sometimes more dangerous ones. So, shutting down unscrupulous pain clinics has shifted people with an existing opioid addiction toward heroin, and heroin is increasingly sold on the street mixed with fentanyl, a significantly more dangerous opioid implicated in the rising rates of overdose deaths.

Our history of top-down, overly restrictive, punitive national policies has also permeated the current addiction treatment system. According to interviewees, patient-centered care, a hot topic in health care, seems to have barely entered the walls of residential and outpatient addiction clinics. Patients are routinely kicked out of treatment for relapse, leaving them with few options other than street purchases, and they are given limited or no choice in the type of care they receive. As one former drug user recently told me, "Treatment centers often resemble prisons more than health care centers."

Despite rhetorical progress in which politicians and the public increasingly call addiction a "disease," our culture's punitive approach toward addiction continues to limit the availability of evidence-based treatment options and person-centered approaches. Not surprisingly, peer-led support groups of current and former drug users remain the most popular recovery support tool, sometimes feeling like the only bastion of compassion toward people with substance use disorder in a judgmental world. Unfortunately, even those in peer support groups often believe that MAT is just another drug.

2

A STRAINED RELATIONSHIP

Alcoholics Anonymous and Medication-Assisted Treatment

UNLIKE JACKSON, PHIL GREW UP with a mother devoted to his happiness. A hardworking ER nurse, she would describe the dangers of drugs to Phil at the dinner table. She was tired of seeing the same teenagers and young adults frequenting the ER, overdose after overdose, as if on a hamster wheel of opioids. She thanked God that her son was not one of those kids. Like many parents, she would soon have a rude awakening.

Ever since his dad died of a heart attack when Phil was only fifteen, Phil had felt an intractable void. Awkward and shy as a teenager, he turned into a cloistered introvert as a college freshman. Living at home with his mother to save money, he rarely left the confines of his room except to attend class. His life felt purposeless and empty. He used alcohol and weed to alleviate boredom but found that he didn't much like either. Phil then tried the oxycodone in his mother's medicine cabinet, fully aware of the dangers. A doctor had prescribed the medication for her following nasal surgery, but she had used only a few pills and failed to discard the others. Phil wasn't exactly looking to get high; he just wanted to see what the medication did for people. Why were they so obsessed with it? Swallowing it, Phil didn't see the big deal. But snorting it, he quickly discovered the answer. Oxycodone made him feel numb and relaxed, two feelings he had strived for since he was fifteen: "It was just like a light bulb went off and I thought, this is great. I could function, and I could still go to school while doing it because I didn't smell like alcohol or weed. It was the answer to all my problems. I could talk to women. I felt better about myself. It was just like a cure-all."

But rather than closing a hole in his life, oxycodone ripped open new ones. Classes started to feel more pointless than ever, so he stopped going. He dropped out of school and spent his days playing video games. Other than his local drug dealers, he had no friends. To support his drug use, Phil regularly stole money from his mother, something she was too busy and too trusting to notice. When she finally did notice, she kicked him out, believing the tough road would be therapeutic. A year passed before Phil was tired of being sick and couch surfing. He contacted his mother, telling her he was ready to stop using. He admitted he needed help. There began a winding journey through abstinence-only rehab centers, support groups, counseling, and buprenorphine treatment. Fortunately for Phil, various factors outside of his control have helped him along the way: his mother's great health insurance through her hospital job, the recently enacted Affordable Care Act policy allowing him to stay on her insurance until age twenty-six, and his urban location with a variety of treatment options. In retrospect, Phil was luckier than most. Even so, the journey has been hard and sometimes he has felt like giving up. Looking back, Phil feels that two tools have helped him the most on his path toward recovery: Alcoholics Anonymous and buprenorphine. But the relationship between these two recovery methods has been less than cordial.

PHIL HAS PARTICIPATED in AA meetings ever since his first stint in rehab. In fact, daily AA meetings were a required component of that program, which took place in a facility affiliated with his mother's hospital. Every evening after dinner, Phil's cohort would gather on chairs positioned in a circle in a meeting room with motivational messages plastered on an otherwise empty white wall. The meeting always began with the Serenity Prayer: "God, grant me the serenity to accept the things I cannot change, courage to change the things I can, and wisdom to know the difference." Next, whoever chose the chair with a laminated green paper would read out loud the rules of the program, called the "traditions," after which the person seated on the chair with the laminated red paper would read out loud the twelve steps.

The chairperson of the meeting, an alternating volunteer position, then introduced himself or herself and shared any announcements. Then the chairperson would ask if this was the first day of anyone's sobriety, after which he or she distributed plastic chips resembling coins indicating other people's progress: one month of sobriety, two months of sobriety, and so forth. Finally, the chairperson would introduce the meeting's topic, typically one of the steps, and anyone who had something to say could jump in, starting with an introduction of himself or herself as "an alcoholic" or "an addict," since the rehab center catered to people recovering from any type of drug.

At first Phil didn't care much for the meetings, but he soon began to enjoy hearing the perspectives of a wide range of people, many of who looked nothing like him but had had similar experiences. Unlike formal counseling sessions, the AA meetings did not have a professional in charge; the group was for peers by peers. But AA meetings were also the foundation of the group counseling offered by the center that was led by professionals, with topics of discussion almost always focused on the twelve steps of AA. Even the reading material available in the bedrooms and common areas was overwhelmingly twelve-step literature.

At the end of the twenty-eight-day residential program, Phil's case manager sat Phil and his mother down for a final talk. The case manager looked Phil squarely in the face and announced, "We have given you the tools for recovery. You have all you need. What you do now is up to you." She then strongly recommended that Phil attend Alcoholics Anonymous or Narcotics Anonymous (NA) daily in the community to stay in recovery. She gave Phil a pamphlet with meeting times and locations. As they drove away from the facility, Phil and his mother felt optimistic. After all, Phil now had the tools for recovery. What could possibly go wrong?

Phil moved back in with his mother. He was neither in school nor working. Recovery was intentionally his full-time focus. He attended AA meetings daily in a nearby Baptist church. He read AA literature at home. He searched the internet for college programs. His mother even joined Phil for "open" AA meetings, meaning meetings open to people not in recovery. She was pleased with Phil's progress. He had a sponsor with whom he met regularly for coffee and to watch comedy films.

But within a few months, Phil's mother started getting pangs of anxiety. They were caused by little things, such as seeing Phil falling asleep randomly or scratching himself. Unbeknownst to her, Phil had started using again only a few weeks after being released from rehab—small amounts at first, allowing him to hide the behavior—but like before, the habit quickly escalated. Looking back, he doesn't really know why he relapsed, other than he still had physical and psychological cravings and thought about getting high daily.

Phil's mother confronted her son and threatened to kick him out of the spare bedroom if he didn't stop using opioids. Unlike a year ago, Phil was eager to get help. He had plans for college. He did not want to resume couch surfing. So, he asked his mother to send him to rehab again, and once more she agreed. Like a *Twilight Zone* episode, history repeated itself. Phil returned to the same hospital-affiliated rehab center. Combined, insurance and his mother paid close to $30,000.

Trapped inside the facility, he did great. He brushed up on the tools for recovery. He rekindled his motivation to stay drug-free. As before, he returned home and resumed daily AA meetings. He once more met regularly with his sponsor. Then one evening Phil's mom called home from work to check in and heard a stream of incongruous sentences and gibberish on the other end of the line. There was no doubt—he was using yet again. Worried that he was at risk of overdose, she rushed home. She would have preferred to call an ambulance, but she didn't want the police showing up with the paramedics. She did not want her son going to jail and ruining any chances for his future. Despite its seeming failures, the rehab center had at least taught them that addiction was a disease that could be treated.

In the ER that night, a physician named Dr. Aman was making rounds, temporarily replacing another physician who could not attend work that day. Dr. Aman's son was in recovery from heroin addiction through a medication called Suboxone. The fortuitousness of this chance meeting continues to strike Phil as one of those weird coincidences that changes your life. Dr. Aman recommended that Phil start taking Suboxone, although Dr. Aman could not prescribe it himself, at least not more than a few days' worth. Phil would need to find a different, regular prescriber. Phil had heard of Suboxone, but AA participants and the rehab center had taught him that Suboxone was just another drug, and that if he took it, he would not be truly sober. He knew his drug dealer sold it, though at a higher price than other substances, seemingly confirming the rehab center's and AA members' beliefs. As a result, Phil had never before seriously considered it a recovery option.

His mother Googled "Suboxone prescriber" and found a few names. No office was accepting new patients; some said they were simply no longer prescribing Suboxone. Finally, she discreetly asked some colleagues at work and got the name of a local prescriber accepting new patients. In one week Phil would have his first appointment. In the meantime, Phil restarted AA yet again. He is pretty sure that without AA and his sponsor, he would have started using oxycodone during the weeklong gap before starting buprenorphine.

EVEN THOUGH AA DOESN'T SEEM to help him with cravings or withdrawal, it does give Phil a powerful sense of community. Seeing others in long-term recovery has repeatedly inspired him to continue his own journey. Maybe there is light at the end of the tunnel. Phil explained that prior to attending support groups, "I felt so alone and so isolated . . . but when I started going to these meetings, I started hearing other people sharing their stories and it was like seventy to eighty percent of their experience was my experience. It didn't matter if they were a rich black woman, poor black woman, orphan, male, female. It didn't matter where they were coming from; they had so much in common with me, and I started to feel this sense of kinship. And I was able to talk about things that I never talked about to anybody else because there was this understanding and this safe space."

Nevertheless, the combination of AA and buprenorphine has not been easy. When Phil started buprenorphine treatment, his relapses decreased significantly in frequency and intensity, and then they finally stopped. He last misused an opioid two years ago. Today he continues daily buprenorphine treatment and considers himself both sober and in recovery. Unfortunately, others in his AA group do not. Or at least Phil thinks they would not; he has never actually told them about his buprenorphine treatment because of the sprinkling of derogatory comments he hears from time to time. Only Phil's current and previous sponsors know.

Phil's previous sponsor had suggested stopping buprenorphine, but the medication was keeping cravings and withdrawal symptoms at bay, so Phil ignored the advice and eventually found a different sponsor. His latest sponsor is more open to buprenorphine but conversations about the medication remain awkward, as if it is a taboo topic. So Phil usually doesn't mention it. Even if people in AA were to view the medication as helpful, Phil explained, they would still consider it just a Band-Aid or a crutch—not exactly something to be proud of. But Phil is proud of himself; two years is a long time to not misuse drugs, especially when drugs were once the only thing that brought him happiness. Without withdrawal symptoms and cravings, he can focus on his college degree and his relationship with his girlfriend.

Not discussing buprenorphine treatment during group meetings feels uncomfortable. Phil wishes he could discuss it openly. After all, AA teaches you to be honest with yourself and others. I ask Phil how deep the feelings against medication-assisted treatment run in the local AA community. Pretty deep, he thinks, because even his current buprenorphine-prescribing doctor warned him about the stigma he might experience in AA. Nevertheless, she advised Phil to continue twelve-step group participation. She suggested that hiding his buprenorphine treatment status was no big deal: "You don't tell your group about antibiotics you are on, do you? So why should you tell them about your buprenorphine treatment?" But Phil thinks it is relevant. AA is supposed to support you in your recovery through narrative sharing and identity building. And he cannot fully participate in the group without sharing his own recovery story, which involves buprenorphine.

I ask Phil why he continues attending twelve-step meetings. He responds that both buprenorphine and AA are central to his recovery in their own way. AA offers something that buprenorphine cannot offer: practical approaches to living a life that for him, as for many other people in recovery, has been traumatic and chaotic. He gives the following example, "So [AA is] always [emphasizing] taking care of my side of the street. If I'm getting mad about something, it's because of me, not because of what the other person did. There's something inside of me that's making me upset and I need to address [that], not the other person. I can't control anything other than my reaction. Those sorts of things, which are very simple and sound very simple, were just [foreign] to me. You know? . . . That's when I talk about sobriety versus being dry. That's what I'm talking about and that's when I say there needs to be some kind of treatment other than just the chemical side of it."

MILLIONS OF AMERICANS believe that twelve-step support groups have improved their physical, psychological, and spiritual health, and significant research evidence supports this conclusion.[100] But twelve-step support groups, such as Alcoholics Anonymous and Narcotics Anonymous, have a complex relationship with MAT. And MAT has a significantly stronger evidence base for managing opioid use disorder than do behavioral methods such as counseling and support groups.[101]

Twelve-step support groups are America's best known and most widely used addiction management tool.[102] They are the foundation of over half of America's publicly funded addiction treatment centers.[103] Twelve-step participation is routinely mandated as treatment within the criminal justice system[104] and even as discipline by professional medical and legal organizations.[105,106] In much of the United States, twelve-step support groups and treatment centers based on the twelve steps are the only available options for people with substance use disorders, making it almost certain that a person in treatment will be exposed to them.[107] Broadly speaking, this prominence has resulted in an expectation that anyone with a substance use disorder follow the same formula, even though many people disagree with the twelve steps or find them unhelpful. Most concerning, though, is that many twelve-step groups promote an abstinence-only treatment philosophy: the idea that addiction treatment should be medication-free. Nevertheless, people subscribing to MAT may still want to attend AA or NA meetings or may be required to do so by their treatment center or the criminal justice system. Furthermore, people's perceptions of MAT, including whether or not they seek MAT, are likely influenced by twelve-step philosophy. Therefore, to understand the current addiction treatment landscape, including MAT stigma and other barriers to MAT adoption, one must understand twelve-step groups. Let's start with the most common one: AA.

ALCOHOLICS ANONYMOUS is the prototypical twelve-step group on which other twelve-step groups are based. Bill Wilson cofounded

AA in the 1930s after a series of life-changing events. While institutionalized for the fourth time for alcoholism, Bill W., as he came to be known, had a spiritual awakening. Also while institutionalized, he encountered a neurologist who claimed that alcohol addiction was an allergy to alcohol. If you could not stop at one drink, then you had the allergy. People without the allergy, on the other hand, could stop drinking whenever they wanted. This conceptualization of addiction convinced Bill W. that alcoholism was a disease rather than a mark of immorality or insufficient willpower. At the time, the disease concept was hardly mainstream. Some wealthy urbanites pursued psychoanalysis in private psychiatrist offices,[35] but even psychoanalysts claimed that addiction was a character flaw resulting from immaturity and requiring personality transformation.[35]

Following detoxification, Bill W. went on a business trip to Akron, Ohio, where he once more felt the uncontrollable urge to drink. At the same time, he felt a strong impulse to speak to another person with alcohol addiction. He contacted a clergyman at random and asked to be connected to a local alcoholic. The clergyman connected Bill W. with Dr. Bob Smith, a proctologist. The two men met and spent hours discussing their urge to drink and ways to overcome the urge. The experience of storytelling and mutual support gave them both psychological relief and stopped them from hitting the bottle. Soon the two men began searching for others with whom to share their stories, forming new personal identities in the story-sharing process.[35]

The first regular story-sharing group met as part of the Oxford Group, an evangelical Protestant organization. But the direct association with the Oxford Group was short-lived, as Bill W. and Dr. Bob wanted a spiritual rather than a religious group identity, fearing that the latter would deter participation. They formed their own group, which eventually became known as Alcoholics Anonymous, or AA. Nevertheless, AA remained strongly influenced by the beliefs of the Oxford Group and its founder, Frank Buchman.

Buchman, a Lutheran minister, had preached against worldliness and the idea that man could achieve happiness through personal achievement, riches, or fame. He especially abhorred the concept of the self-made, middle-class man aspiring to wealth and success, which he called an American "spiritual sickness." Instead, Buchman argued for "spiritual surgery" consisting of complete surrender to God as understood through the teachings of Jesus Christ and reorientation of one's life around honesty, purity, unselfishness, and love.[108] Only through such surrender could man truly be happy and at peace.

Bill W. combined these basic spiritual concepts from the Oxford Group, though stripped of their explicit religious connotations, with the belief that alcohol addiction was a disease. The result was the twelve steps to recovery: a progression of spiritual, moral, and practical steps for daily living and a recipe to prevent one from drinking. The steps were fodder for discussion during AA group meetings, but each individual member was ultimately responsible for working through the steps on his or her own with the help of a sponsor. The sponsor was another AA member who provided emotional and practical support.[109]

AA's twelve steps, which have been adopted in similar form by other twelve-step groups, are as follows:

1. We admitted we were powerless over alcohol—that our lives had become unmanageable.
2. Came to believe that a Power greater than ourselves could restore us to sanity.
3. Made a decision to turn our will and our lives over to the care of God *as we understood Him*.
4. Made a searching and fearless moral inventory of ourselves.
5. Admitted to God, to ourselves, and to another human being the exact nature of our wrongs.
6. Were entirely ready to have God remove all these defects of character.

7. Humbly asked Him to remove our shortcomings.
8. Made a list of all persons we had harmed, and became willing to make amends to them all.
9. Made direct amends to such people wherever possible, except when to do so would injure them or others.
10. Continued to take personal inventory and when we were wrong promptly admitted it.
11. Sought through prayer and meditation to improve our conscious contact with God *as we understood Him*, praying only for knowledge of His will for us and the power to carry that out.
12. Having had a spiritual awakening as the result of these steps, we tried to carry this message to alcoholics, and to practice these principles in all our affairs.[110]

Within thirty years of Bill W. and Dr. Bob's first meeting, AA became the primary alcohol treatment mechanism in 88 percent of state hospitals. In 1979, sociologist Robert Tournier wrote that AA's assumptions about addiction and addiction treatment had "virtually been accepted as fact by most of the field."[111] A spiritually based, nonprofessional support group had become the dominant treatment method for addiction in an increasingly medicalized world. Some called it the most successful social movement in the history of America. Soon AA's program would be applied to other addictions, ranging from drug addiction to eating disorders to gambling addiction. Narcotics Anonymous took the twelve steps and applied them to people recovering from drugs, though many people whom I have interviewed go to AA despite having nonalcohol drug problems. AA and NA still remain the most popular twelve-step groups, with an estimated 1.2 million members[112] and 250,000 members[113] in the United States, respectively, though accurate numbers are difficult to come by given members' anonymity. An estimated 6–9 percent of the US adult population has at one time or another attended a twelve-step meeting.[113,114]

Like many Americans, Phil's understanding of his own addiction is strongly influenced by AA tenets: "As I understand addiction, it's a disease that is progressive and fatal, and I'm never going to be cured, so I don't think there's ever going to be a point where I can stop going to meetings and then maybe have a drink here or there. . . . It doesn't matter what kind of chemicals I'm taking at that point if I'm not really trying to improve myself, then I'm not going to get any benefit from it in the long run." His quote is rich with common AA teachings: one must attend AA meetings indefinitely to prevent relapse; AA is about self-improvement, not just ending drinking; and addiction will cause death if not managed. The idea that one drink will lead to complete chaos is consistent with AA's original understanding of addiction as an allergy to a substance, an allergy requiring complete abstinence.

AA and NA are not treatment per se. In fact, they do not even refer to themselves as treatment. But they can be misunderstood as such given the frequency with which they are used in treatment centers. Instead, they are peer-led mutual support groups available in the community at no cost. They are not professional or clinical services. However, many treatment centers provide "twelve-step facilitation therapy" in which counselors prepare people for twelve-step groups in the community, further confusing the public as to the "treatment" status of AA and NA.

That said, the twelve steps are about far more than stopping drug or alcohol use. Only the first of the twelve steps directly relates to substances. The remaining steps are about living life in general. Phil says, "I think the twelve steps are not about the drug side; they're more about the spiritual or the mental [psychological] well-being of the person. I think anybody would benefit from that particular program. It just happened to be a bunch of alcoholics who hit on this. And I think if they weren't alcoholics, it probably would be some kind of cult." The twelve steps' broad focus on spirituality, morality, and daily habits can complement MAT's focus on physical health, just as exercise and healthy diet can complement insulin treatment in diabetes care.

The broad twelve-step perspective may explain the method's influence on so many lives, especially when one considers social cohesion and spirituality as recovery end points, rather than the mere absence of drugs on urine screens.[115] For example, the American Society of Addiction Medicine believes the combination of medications and therapy is the best treatment for opioid use disorder, but it also describes twelve-step support groups as improving social interconnectedness with others, boosting spirituality, and encouraging help-seeking behaviors.[116]

Unfortunately, despite these benefits, AA and NA are associated with an abstinence-only philosophy in treatment centers and among counselors. For example, one-third of centers in a nationally representative 2011 study cited abstinence-only ideology as a barrier to MAT, including the perception that MAT was "just another drug," and twelve-step philosophy was associated with this abstinence-only ideology.[117] Studies show that counselors who oppose MAT are particularly likely to have adopted a twelve-step philosophy.[118,119]

Abstinence-only treatment centers may exhibit their anti-medication ideology in various ways. Many explicitly prohibit clients from starting MAT or continuing MAT previously begun outside of the treatment center. Other treatment centers only allow MAT for detoxification rather than for long-term maintenance, or they only allow MAT at a low dose. Yet longer-term, higher-dose MAT is associated with better opioid relapse prevention, decreased overdose rates, and greater adherence to HIV/AIDS medications.[17,120,121] These anti-MAT attitudes are influenced by treatment centers' reliance on twelve-step philosophy, which they interpret as prohibiting MAT, especially buprenorphine and methadone.

In addition to contributing to MAT stigma in treatment centers, twelve-step groups have also directly stigmatized their own members in the community who use MAT. This very stigma led to the creation of Methadone Anonymous as an alternative to AA and NA, though this alternative group is only available in a few areas. Methadone Anonymous follows essentially the same twelve steps but explicitly accepts people undergoing methadone treatment. In step one, the group states, "We admitted we were powerless over illicit drugs, including alcohol." By adding the word "illicit," the group hopes to clarify that utilizing a medication properly as prescribed by a physician is not a problem, because it is licit.[122]

In its most recent pamphlet on the topic, *Narcotics Anonymous and Persons Receiving Medication-Assisted Treatment* (2016),[123] NA has dialed back the anti-MAT tone found in some of its previous publications (such as Bulletin #29 from 1996)[124] and are encouraging a judgment-free atmosphere to attract newcomers. But even still, NA headquarters reiterates individual NA groups' freedom to bar people utilizing MAT from full participation: "Some NA meetings make no distinction as to whether those receiving medication to treat addiction may share in a meeting, while other NA meetings limit the participation of those who are taking this type of medication. Each group is free to make its own decision on recovery meeting participation and involvement in group services for those receiving medication assistance for drug addiction."[123]

Problematically, NA also continues to identify people recovering through MAT as not being "clean." For example, they state, "Clean in NA typically refers to being free of all drugs, or abstinent. However, an addict who is not clean is free to attend meetings. . . . Sometimes people come to NA meetings while still using drugs, detoxing from drugs, or on drug replacement therapy. Regardless of what you may be taking when you first come to NA, you are welcome."[123] Clearly, people on "replacement therapy," a term referring to buprenorphine or methadone, are still not clean but rather in the same category as those misusing drugs or detoxing from illicit drugs. Explaining that it takes some people longer to get clean than others, the 2016 publication also describes a former methadone patient: "He wanted what he saw in the rooms of Narcotics Anonymous but was afraid of returning to his old life if he quit methadone. For ten months, he went to meetings every day—and finally he got clean."[123] Again, this quote implies the man was not clean until he stopped his methadone treatment.

One can easily imagine the disappointment and cognitive dissonance experienced by a person who has not misused opioids for a year being told that they are not really clean, sober, or in recovery—that there is no meaningful difference between receiving MAT as prescribed with no euphoria and using heroin daily to get high. Such stigma can be especially harmful for a population that has already experienced significant social isolation and psychological trauma.[125] Stan, another of my interviewees who is undergoing methadone treatment, thinks the nonjudgmental language of AA and NA literature is meaningless without full participation for people utilizing MAT. He says, "And of course, the twelve-step program is going to say it is okay for you to go to meetings. You could go to the meetings where you can't talk. You can't open your mouth, which is completely ridiculous and upsets me just thinking about that right now."

How common is MAT stigma within twelve-step groups? There has never been a national survey of twelve-step group members' opinions on MAT, but smaller studies and my own qualitative research suggest that stigma is deeply entrenched in AA and NA groups. In a recent study of over 250 twelve-step members undergoing methadone treatment, one quarter reported serious problems related to their methadone status.[126] Problems included hearing negative comments about methadone, pressure to reduce or stop methadone, being unable to speak at a meeting or hold a position in the meeting, and being unable to act as a sponsor. In the study, approximately 40 percent of people undergoing methadone treatment kept their status hidden from the support group. Interestingly, despite the stigma, a majority found twelve-step groups helpful to their own recovery, but two-thirds did not recommend twelve-step referrals for others treated with methadone.[126]

A similar study of buprenorphine patients in twelve-step groups found that a third of them did not reveal their treatment status to their groups or sponsors for fear of being stigmatized.[125] Another study found that people coparticipating in buprenorphine treatment and twelve-step groups frequently failed to consider their time on buprenorphine as "clean time." Some participants started viewing buprenorphine as a "crutch," causing them to want to discontinue treatment early.[127] Early discontinuation is dangerous; rates of relapse after buprenorphine discontinuation are consistently 50 percent across studies.[128] Julie, a young woman in Florida, has had a similar experience: "I was very pro-MAT, and I always stayed pro-MAT. But to be completely honest with you, I went to [AA] meetings that saved me and everything, and at some point I became anti-MAT. I still accepted everyone that came into the meeting, but I definitely started forming a negative connotation toward it my first year in recovery until I started educating myself more again. I don't want to say I was almost brainwashed, but I just really wanted people to like me." Eventually Julie started standing up for participants at her meetings undergoing MAT and then started an alternative local support group for those who felt rejected by AA.

So why do so many twelve-step groups and abstinence-only treatment centers stigmatize MAT? Is it possible that twelve-step groups and MAT can be effectively combined for some people, ending the battle between these recovery methods once and for all? Why can't everyone just get along?

PHIL DOES NOT BELIEVE he would be here today without both MAT and AA in his life. He says they are two important recovery tools that are largely misunderstood, both inside and outside of the recovery community. He is tired of having to explain to friends, family, and treatment providers that MAT is not just another drug and that AA is not just some religious cult. But for my sake, I ask him to walk me through his thought process. What exactly is recovery and can both MAT and AA fit in? Why does it seem like there is a battle between them?

According to Phil and others whom I have interviewed, recovery is an ambiguous concept, sometimes defined as the process of creating a meaningful life or improving one's quality of life. With such a loose definition, recovery is difficult to measure empirically, especially as one person's definition of a meaningful life may differ from another's. Measuring recovery is further complicated by it being *both* a process and a destination. You can be in recovery even if you relapse, so long as you are still generally on the path toward improving your own life according to your own goals. If this makes recovery sound mushy and kind of boundaryless, that's because it is.

The concept of recovery is broad enough to include personal self-improvement goals ranging from physical health to employment, housing, spiritual health, mental health, family life, and social life. MAT clearly fits into the recovery model, as it improves physical health. Furthermore, by stabilizing one's life, MAT can improve employment, family life, social life, and the progress of other personal goals. Likewise, twelve-step groups also fit within the recovery model by improving mental health, spiritual health, and social life.

But even though the concept of recovery is wide enough to encompass both twelve-step groups and MAT, treatment centers and support group meetings often present them as opposing forces—as if MAT prevents recovery while twelve-step groups further it. This misconception is largely due to a basic misunderstanding of the meanings of recovery, sobriety, treatment, physical dependence, and addiction.

Recovery, when viewed as a destination, incorporates a broad spectrum of end points that can include abstinence from all drugs but also everything from harm reduction (using drugs in a less dangerous manner than before) to an enhanced mental state, improved social networks, or development of healthy habits. Only the person in recovery can answer the question "Are you in recovery?" because the definition is so individualized. Nevertheless, compared to chaotic or constant drug use without harm reduction measures, recovery is almost certainly a place of better health outcomes.

Sobriety, in contrast, is the mere abstinence from drugs to which you are addicted. Sobriety presents a dichotomy rather than a spectrum: either you are using drugs to which you are addicted or you are completely sober. You are never "kind of sober" or "almost sober." In contrast, recovery is a much more flexible concept allowing for different stages of change. It is thus more pragmatic and realistic. For example, you cannot be sober if you used heroin this morning, but you could still be in recovery if you experienced a momentary relapse that you are already taking steps to address. As a process, recovery can include professional treatment such as MAT. But recovery can also include other life-enhancing tools, ranging from religion to support groups. Phil explained it to me this way: "Treatment, I've been in treatment, but I want to be in recovery . . . and again, treatment's something you can force somebody into and recovery isn't."

Recovery, sobriety, and treatment are all related to the concept of drug addiction. Simply put, drug addiction is the *compulsive use* of a substance resulting in an overwhelmingly *negative impact* on one's life. The negative impact on one's life is critical to the definition or else breathing oxygen would be considered an addiction simply because it is compulsive. Likewise, just because someone is taking opioids regularly and exhibits withdrawal symptoms or tolerance does not mean they have an addiction, even if their body is physically dependent. Someone prescribed opioids for pain could experience a generally positive impact from finally being able to get out of bed and attend work or play with their children. On the other hand, someone with an opioid addiction experiences a generally negative impact from opioids. For example, the compulsive opioid use causes their marriage to crumble and their bank account to be drained.

Methadone and buprenorphine are opioids that activate the opioid receptors in the brain, so people taking methadone or buprenorphine as addiction treatment will almost certainly become physically dependent on the medications. But they are not addicted to the medications if the overall impact on their life is *positive*. And we know from decades of studies that buprenorphine and methadone promote a more stable life for people with opioid addiction, letting them refocus on work, their families, and other responsibilities. Their lives often feel more meaningful too because they are not living merely for the next high. Since their cravings and withdrawal symptoms are controlled, they might even go hours, days, or weeks without thinking about misusing drugs. And they are also significantly less likely to die of an overdose[24,101,129–133]—surely a net positive. So, when abstinence-only treatment centers and twelve-step groups call MAT "just another drug" or "just another addiction," they are really confusing physical dependence with addiction.

If the net-effect of MAT on someone's life is positive, then MAT is promoting recovery, especially when one considers such wide-reaching recovery goals as life stability. But how can you be sober if you have an opioid—any opioid—in your system? Isn't sobriety, after all, the absence of drugs? Not entirely. Sobriety is the absence of drugs *to which you are addicted*. That is why a person with cancer pain taking hydrocodone as prescribed for pain management is sober: he is not compulsively taking it despite negative consequences. Will he experience physical withdrawal symptoms if the hydrocodone is terminated abruptly? Probably. He has also likely reached a tolerance threshold. But again, this is physical dependence, not addiction. Likewise, someone taking methadone or buprenorphine as prescribed for addiction treatment without negative consequences is sober. If anything, they are taking a medication with overwhelmingly positive consequences, such as physiological stability due to elimination of cravings and withdrawal symptoms.

The way in which twelve-step groups limit the definition of recovery can cause confusion, stigma, and shame. Stan, who was concurrently undergoing buprenorphine treatment and participating in AA in North Carolina explained, "There were some years [in AA] where I was told that I had never experienced real recovery because my only amount of sobriety was on [Suboxone]. And I bought into [it], I believed it as well. I've kind of gone through all the different stages of AA and views on [Suboxone]. Like I've looked down on it myself, I've done it and been frowned upon. I guess the most supportive period I got in AA while on [Suboxone] was that first sponsor who said, 'I wish you'd get off of it, but you can still work the steps.'"

I asked Stan how such statements made him feel. I heard the frustration in his voice as he responded, "I knew that my life on Suboxone looks a hell of a lot different than my life in chaotic heroin drug use. Like I'm not being homeless, getting arrested, all the really horrible things that can happen in drug use. So, when they say, 'oh, that's not recovery,' well Suboxone was nothing like heroin for me. The whole time in the program, people tell you, 'Take what you want, leave the rest' but at the same time they're saying, 'Your thinking got you here, so you need to listen to us.' And you can have a lot of cognitive dissonance where you just make it up for yourself."

AA WAS INSTRUMENTAL in catalyzing the recovery movement, so if any group should have an accurate understanding of recovery, it should be AA. It has always viewed drug use as nested within the broader context of one's daily habits, spirituality, and social support. Unfortunately, some AA and NA groups have squeezed MAT out of their recovery definition, despite the fact that AA literature refers medical issues to physicians rather than support groups. But according to many people in AA and NA whom I have interviewed, there is no technical reason why AA and NA could not incorporate MAT into their definitions of recovery. It would require changing culture at the group level and some pro-MAT statements from AA and NA headquarters. And according to an interview with Vincent P. Dole, the famous methadone researcher, Bill W. did not oppose methadone. In fact, Bill W. encouraged Dole to research a medication that would do for alcohol addiction what methadone does for opioid addiction.[134]

Even when twelve-step participants, counselors, or treatment centers understand the potential benefits of MAT, they are sometimes concerned that MAT will push people away from other recovery methods, such as support groups or counseling. For example, during my presentations, counselors frequently ask, "But won't people who take medication just stop coming to counseling, harming their overall recovery?" A cynical person might view these attitudes as mere self-preservation, but many treatment providers sincerely believe that MAT leaves little room for anything else. I've also heard the concern phrased, "Since taking medication is so easy, why would anyone do the hard work of the twelve steps or counseling?"

When asked whether he would sponsor someone in AA taking Suboxone, Jake, a long-term AA adherent with an abstinence-only philosophy, responded, "I'm not going to cosign that because in that case you're basically using [Suboxone] as your Higher Power—that's what's keeping you from shooting dope. . . . It makes people just comfortable enough to where they don't really need to do the steps. Anybody can go to a meeting, anybody can go to the gym, but are you actually lifting weights?" As Jake's comment reveals, some AA members fear that Suboxone will prevent one from working through the steps or having a relationship with a Higher Power, as if full AA participation rather than recovery is the end goal. It's like worrying that a diabetic will not watch their diet or exercise if you offer them insulin, so maybe we should just keep the insulin away.

In fact, later in his interview, Jake suggested that people on MAT should be welcome at AA meetings because the exposure to AA principles might lead them to quit MAT and follow AA exclusively. This is not acceptance of MAT. It's like an evangelical church telling homosexuals that they are welcome, not because the church approves of homosexuality, but because by packing the pews with homosexuals, the church has the opportunity to show them how to lead "godly" lives instead. As Jake explains, "Whether they're under the influence of MAT or not, I think the seeds still get planted regardless. I've got a friend that used to go to meetings in Boston drunk every week. He's been sober twelve years now."

Ironically, MAT likely promotes counseling and support group attendance, perhaps because people whose cravings and withdrawal symptoms are controlled can better focus on their social and psychological problems.[130] It's really common sense, a version of Maslow's hierarchy in which people's basic physiological needs must be addressed before they can focus on their psychological needs. As Alyssa, a former sex worker in the Midwest, explained to me, "To this day, I credit being alive to Suboxone, because what the Suboxone did for me was I was able to focus on what was being said in [AA] meetings and to listen to the message of recovery because I wasn't constantly thinking about my physical symptoms because they were not present. I wasn't craving. I felt like how I imagined normal people feel when they wake up." It gave her the space to do the emotional work of recovery, to examine the underlying reasons for her drug use. She calls buprenorphine the "legs of a chair," providing the stability on which to build recovery.

But despite having attended meetings daily and sponsoring people, and even being a circuit speaker for AA, Alyssa was very careful to whom she revealed her Suboxone treatment. At one meeting, one of the "hard-core" AA participants told her, "You're not really in recovery," even though she was back in school and no longer selling sex for drugs or sleeping in her car. She was no longer getting high. In fact, everything in her life had changed for the better. But even her fiancé, whom she met in AA, pressured her to quit Suboxone, telling her it was a condition of them getting married. The marriage lasted only one year.

Eventually the anti-MAT stigma became too much, and there were other issues with her local AA groups as well. Some of the older men were predatory toward younger women. Plus, she'd never had problems with alcohol and she liked to have a glass of wine with dinner, something the group, of course, opposed. So even though Alyssa had not misused opioids for years, between Suboxone treatment and drinks with dinner she was never allowed to claim "clean time."

Today, Alyssa no longer attends AA or actively works the steps. But still she says, "I use the principles in my life constantly, about letting go and about recognizing that I'm powerless. And, in fact, what I learned from AA has helped me in every single relationship: work relationships, romantic relationships, relationships with my children . . . it's helped me have more positive interactions with people." She firmly believes that AA is important for many people, especially those seeking a new social network and the tools to lead a fulfilling life after quitting drugs or alcohol. Yet she admits it's not for everyone.

Also, quitting AA was hard at first. Alyssa missed the camaraderie. It was like axing her whole social network, including a very robust dating scene, sometimes jokingly referred to as the "thirteenth step." But over the last few years, she has found camaraderie elsewhere—in the local harm reduction coalition.

I have spent much time speaking with two pillars of the national harm reduction community, Chris Abert in the Midwest and Justin Kunzelman in the Southeast, learning how harm reduction saves lives, a fact supported by a wide variety of studies.[50,135,136] Harm reduction is an approach to treatment in which you meet people where they are at, offer them a variety of evidence-based recovery tools, and help them make and meet their own goals. It is the opposite of the one-size-fits-all abstinence-only treatment on which US addiction care has been based for decades. Harm reduction philosophy says you can quit heroin but still have a beer; you can be in buprenorphine treatment and still consider yourself sober. And if you aren't ready to quit heroin, harm reductionists will at least give you the tools to stay safe until you are ready. These tools might include clean needles through a syringe exchange program, so you don't get HIV/AIDS; supervised heroin injection sites with drug quality tests, so you don't accidently overdose when heroin is laced with elephant tranquilizer; and take-home naloxone, so your loved one or friend can give you an antidote if you overdose. A key harm reduction phrase is "You can't recover if you're dead." And once you are ready to recover, harm reductionists will connect you to resources, including MAT.

In her current volunteer work, Alyssa helps local sex workers: a vulnerable group that faces tremendous stigma and violence and is often plagued with opioid addiction. Before recovering, Alyssa would spend fifteen minutes in the backseat of local politicians' cars for $300, thus funding her heroin purchases. Now she teaches sex workers harm reduction practices she wishes she had known all those years ago—such as not using water from the toilet to distill your drugs.

Eventually, after her physiological opioid cravings and withdrawal symptoms stopped, Alyssa transitioned off buprenorphine. Nevertheless, she wants to understand why she used drugs for so many years. She thinks it has something to do with her childhood trauma and history of low self-esteem, for which she has been receiving mental health therapy. She explained, "When my sister takes an opiate, she vomits and can't stay awake. I take an opiate and it's like cocaine for me—I'm awake and I want to chat, I want to talk and I want to do things and I want to play the piano and then I want to go run a marathon, and I feel like I've been held underwater my whole life and somebody finally let me up to breathe, and I'm just taking my first breath. That's what it always felt like to me. And when people asked me what it's like to do heroin, I'm like, 'God, don't ever do it because it's the best thing I've ever felt in my whole life.' But I couldn't sustain it because I had such a dark hole inside of me that I wasn't able to fill. There was no bottom to it. So, for me it was kind of like figuring out how to plug the hole. The hole was trauma and insecurity. And I'm kind of finding my way back from that."

FEW TREATMENT CENTERS offer MAT. When they do, many outpatient and residential addiction treatment centers force patients into twelve-step programs or counseling as a prerequisite or corequirement for MAT. Medication is used as a carrot: if you learn the twelve steps, then we will give you your medication. Of course, I have never seen the reverse: if you take your medicine, we will let you attend counseling or support groups. Numerous practical and ethical problems exist with this coercive treatment approach. In fact, the federal government now recommends against it.[23,28] But let's start with the problem of forcing spirituality onto someone who may not be spiritual in an increasingly secular society.

Like a religion, AA and NA put their trust in a Higher Power and have components of a subculture: their own way of speaking ("My name is John, and I'm an alcoholic"), their own philosophy, and their own traditions (e.g., sitting in a circle, reading the twelve steps with coffee in hand). But Phil, like the vast majority of AA adherents whom I have interviewed, calls AA spiritual rather than religious: "In the beginning, it was heavily, heavily Christian. And there were a couple people involved who really raised a stink about using phrases like 'the Higher Power' or 'God of understanding,' rather than the Judeo-Christian God. And those little differences for me made all the difference. I never would have showed up if it was just a Christian thing."

Phil does not believe in God, so he admits that the Higher Power concept was hard to wrap his head around at first: "That's tough. For a long time, I didn't [buy into it] . . . just 'fake it till you make it.' Then I started saying the collective consciousness of the group is my Higher Power, my sponsors. And it's not a specific person, it's just an institutional, generational knowledge that's sponsor to sponsor, from the very beginning of guys and men and women who have been sober and have found ways to be happy after they were suicidal from their abuse and whatever tragedy happened to them. They found this way by talking to other alcoholics and sharing their experience, and by following these twelve simple steps. And that is still my Higher Power."

Fascinatingly, even though Phil does not believe in God, he prays daily. Why, I asked. "I pray because people that I know that are happy pray. And my sponsors told me to pray. And so I prayed, but I don't believe in a God. If some kind of God wants to reveal itself to me, I'm open to that, but barring any of that, I don't think about it that much, honestly." Basically, Phil goes through the motions without dwelling on exactly how AA works. All he knows is that AA helps him. Yet even he admits that some AA groups adopt an overtly religious tone. He describes meetings that begin with the Lord's Prayer, which makes him feel uncomfortable since he identifies as an agnostic Jew. And Phil is not the first person to tell me about AA meetings in which a Christian prayer is said. Another interviewee described an AA meeting in a state university's clinic where everyone said the Lord's Prayer in a circle while holding hands.

Even if AA is spiritual rather than religious, some people are uncomfortable with any spirituality being used to manage what they perceive as a predominantly medical condition. Megan, whose twenty-six-year-old son, Daniel, is recovering from heroin addiction through the help of methadone and counseling, said Daniel was regularly forced to attend twelve-step programs in rehab centers. She explains, "My son has faith but not traditional faith. . . . He has had to do twelve-step meetings. I just don't know that it's the answer for everyone all the time, and if people are deep in that stuff, if they believe, then I respect that, but I don't think it's the only way. And I guess for me personally, I have a hard time with saying it's a disease and then saying that a religious-based program is what's going to treat it. So, I think there's a place for both, but he needs to be able to have [other] options."

Of course, no problem exists if someone chooses to attend an AA or NA group because of, or in spite of, the group's spiritual components. But it is problematic when treatment centers force spirituality on unwilling participants. And spirituality in addiction treatment centers is difficult to avoid, even though spirituality rarely, if ever, appears as a routine component of treatment for other medical conditions. For example, a 2004 study of nationally representative publicly funded addiction treatment centers, meaning those that received at least 50 percent of their funding from the federal, state, or local government, found that spirituality was more often emphasized than medication. Over 60 percent of those treatment centers had a twelve-step group attendance requirement. And over 50 percent said their center was based on a twelve-step model, with the majority of the remaining centers incorporating the twelve steps in some way.[103]

Even aside from spirituality, some people simply do not relate to the twelve steps or mutual support groups. Even spiritual people don't always find AA or NA helpful. Approximately 40 percent of people who start AA drop out within one year, suggesting that more alternatives are needed.[137] Personality may partly predict who likes and doesn't like twelve-step groups. People with higher "affiliative need," meaning people who are feelings-oriented, are more likely than those with lower affiliative need to participate in AA.[111] People with an external locus of control, meaning those who feel that things happen *to them* rather than *because of* them, may also be more responsive to the twelve steps. In fact, one large survey found that having an external locus of control was the single most powerful predictor of AA affiliation.[107] AA teaches that putting your life in your own hands spells disaster. You have already tried to control your drinking or drug use by "playing God" and it has repeatedly failed.[138] Now it is time to be "not God" and look beyond yourself to a Higher Power, whether that is your support group or Jesus. In this context, taking medication to control your cravings, withdrawal symptoms, and to prevent highs may seem too self-reliant, as if you are once more playing God rather than relying on your Higher Power.

Instead of forcing AA onto clients, treatment centers should try to match recovery methods to clients' individual belief systems. In health care, person-centered care is better care, resulting in greater treatment retention and adherence, which then leads to better health outcomes.[139] Person-centered care has different dimensions, including respecting a person's treatment preferences and values, providing adequate information about his or her health care, providing emotional support, integrating family and significant others in the health care process, providing physical comfort, and aiding transition back into the community.[139] A treatment center that adopts a one-size-fits-all approach or prevents MAT unless you participate in a twelve-step group is not person-centered. Instead, treatment centers should explicitly acknowledge that AA does not work for everyone and offer alternatives. But traditionally, when someone drops out of AA or relapses, the interpretation is that the person did not work the steps, did not have sufficient motivation, or is still in denial about their addiction.[107] The interpretation is rarely: AA did not work for this person.

FORTUNATELY OR UNFORTUNATELY, a top-down change is not possible in AA or NA. They are decentralized organizations with decision-making power held almost entirely at the individual group level. Over time, changes may filter up the food chain, but that can take decades. Therefore, individual support groups must initiate change rather than wait for mandates from the top. They have an obligation to do so. After all, AA and NA are the most widely available help for persons with addiction, both geographically and financially. One study suggests that the acceptance of MAT in twelve-step groups is more likely to begin with buprenorphine than with methadone,[127] so maybe that's where the discussion should begin, given that stigma against methadone is often more pronounced than stigma against buprenorphine. Even if a group is not ready to make a bold statement of support for those undergoing MAT, the group can at least refrain from disparaging the treatment method. After all, a key AA principle is to not directly give advice but rather to teach through storytelling.

Sarah, a regular AA attendee, has taken the bold step of speaking out in favor of MAT at her AA meetings. She proudly explains, "I sponsor people on medication-assisted treatment, which is not really the consensus in AA at this time. A lot of people are kind of closed off to that concept in this area. But I do, and whenever somebody asks me to speak at a meeting, I speak about me sponsoring. I don't really care if it offends someone. Some people may think that's wrong, or me imposing my views, but I have my reasons and I'm really passionate about it." This is not easy to do, as support groups often replace old social networks that once revolved around drug use. Alienating one's key recovery-oriented social network can be a risk to successful recovery.

Stan likewise described how NA affected his beliefs about MAT. He says, "I used to be one of those people that would say that [methadone treatment is not recovery] . . . I turned into the person I hated. I really did. I got that chip on my shoulder, you know, that I'm better . . . I think for a period I thought I was better than everybody else. And look where it ended. I relapsed just as quick as everybody else did." He eventually dealt with the stigma by leaving NA.

In dozens of interviews with people in recovery across many states, almost every interviewee has described serious anti-MAT stigma in twelve-step groups. At the minimum, MAT prescribers should prepare patients for the stigma they may face.[125] They should provide methods for navigating this stigma without necessarily discouraging twelve-step support group participation. They can encourage patients to "shop around," trying different groups. Interviewees frequently tell me that they feel more comfortable in AA than in NA when undergoing MAT, so shopping around should include both types of twelve-step groups. Many AA groups welcome people with drug addiction, not only people with alcohol addiction.

Equally importantly, treatment centers and providers can encourage alternatives to twelve-step groups. Research suggests that twelve-step group effectiveness is closely related to simply changing the drug user's social network by replacing time spent with former drug-using friends.[140] If this is true, then being part of any support group is likely to be helpful, regardless of whether it follows a twelve-step program. Recent studies support this conclusion, demonstrating that non-twelve-step support groups have equivalent outcomes as twelve-step support groups for alcohol addiction, though no study to date has compared outcomes for opioid addiction.[141,142] Alternative groups include LifeRing, SMART Recovery, SOS (Secular Organizations for Sobriety), and Women for Sobriety, to name a few. For example, in contrast to AA's spiritual approach, SMART Recovery uses principles from cognitive behavioral therapy and motivational interviewing, teaching people how to problem-solve and recognize triggers. For those who like the twelve steps but want a support group explicitly open to MAT, they can try Methadone Anonymous or Medication-Assisted Recovery Anonymous.

Unfortunately, twelve-step alternatives are rarely available outside of major metropolitan areas. They are also rarely recommended; addiction treatment centers are four times as likely to recommend twelve-step groups over other support groups, and only a small minority of programs recommend multiple support group options.[143] Counselors who have themselves recovered through twelve-step programs are more likely to refer clients to twelve-step programs, resulting in few recommendations for twelve-step alternatives.[144] Part of the problem lies in the assumption that treatment requires spiritual components. Research does not support this assumption, as belief in a Higher Power does not predict abstinence, even though it does predict twelve-step participation.[141]

At a recent annual American Society of Addiction Medicine conference, one of the preeminent conferences in the world about addiction, I attended a tightly packed presentation called "Combining Medications with 12 Step, Abstinence-Based Treatment for Opioid Use Disorders." Finally, I thought, an attempt to bridge the gap between these two treatments. While the presentation was indeed groundbreaking, I was taken aback by the question-and-answer session. Handed a microphone, I asked, "Shouldn't we be talking about expanding non-twelve-step support groups as well as twelve-step support groups?" The answer, precipitated by audience laughter, was, "If non-twelve-step groups actually worked, they would be more popular, wouldn't they?" And that was the end of that question. Clearly, we still have a long way to go.

IN A NONDESCRIPT STOREFRONT OFFICE, Julie leads a weekly support group called MARA, short for Medication-Assisted Recovery Anonymous. It's a twelve-step peer support group that is a safe space for people undergoing MAT. She explained the local MARA group's humble beginning: "Basically, the common consensus in the area was that these people on medication-assisted treatment really, truly did want to go to twelve-step meetings, for the most part. But they just felt completely out of place or judged. So, my boss and I started doing research, and we found a group that was formed in Virginia. And we basically just printed out the literature and revised it, and we just started having it every Tuesday. We built it, and they came. It started off with just me, my buddy John, who's also in AA with me, and then a kid named Ryan, who is on medication-assisted treatment. And slowly but surely, more people started coming, and now it's been about two months, and it's up to like twenty people, give or take. And it's growing."

How do Julie's MARA meetings compare to local AA meetings? Like in AA, group members sit in a circle, usually with coffee in hand. They share stories of recovery and the pitfalls along the way. In contrast to local AA groups, they openly discuss MAT, including stigma, access problems, and any side effects they experience. They discuss what it's like to start and come off the medications. Even though there is no technical leader of the group, Julie serves as the informal chairperson. If the discussion gets too deep in the medical weeds, such as when participants have questions about medication-to-medication interactions, Julie reminds the participants that they should speak to a physician. But sometimes the discussion isn't about MAT at all. Sometimes it's just about classic twelve-step concepts, such as gratitude or avoiding triggers, except in a space where people utilizing MAT are recognized as truly in recovery.

Unlike local AA meetings, Julie's MARA group spends little time discussing a Higher Power, but no one would shut the topic down if it were brought up. Julie also describes the MARA meetings as more flexible than local AA meetings: "It's a little bit more compassionate than AA meetings. I won't shut anyone down if someone goes off on a tangent. Sometimes in AA, the chairperson will shut it down. I won't. I'll just let someone go, because obviously they needed to say it. And there's no formal correct way. Like in AA, it's almost frowned upon if you don't say, 'Hi. My name is so and so. I'm an alcoholic.' . . . I usually say at MARA meetings, 'Hi. My name's Julie. I'm in recovery.'" In other words, Julie feels this new group offers greater flexibility, allowing people to forgo some of the traditional components of twelve-step groups.

Julie thinks more people are joining her MARA group because anti-MAT stigma is spreading among young adults on social media. She describes anti-MAT memes shared on Facebook recovery groups, making fun of people on buprenorphine or methadone. At the same time, she doesn't put up with "twelve-step bashing" that sometimes creeps into MARA meetings, because ultimately Julie thinks the problem lies not with the twelve steps but rather with the way some AA groups are implementing them. She emphasizes that AA groups should be open to all regardless of their preferred recovery methods. Being open to the newcomer and meeting them where they are at is a fundamental component of the original twelve-step program, as is not judging others. She believes it is completely possible for AA groups to accept MAT and those who use MAT. But in describing local group approaches to MAT, Julie grimaces saying, "They're literally taking the main principle of how the program was built in 1938, and just fucking stepping on it."

But some AA adherents disagree with Julie's beliefs about twelve-step and MAT compatibility, though only a small minority of people whom I have interviewed. For example, discussing buprenorphine and methadone, interviewee Lee explains, "I don't understand why somebody would want to introduce addictive substances to a community that's trying to get off of addictive stuff." While admitting that MAT saves lives and that newcomers on MAT should be welcomed into meetings, he later explains that AA should never accept MAT as a recovery method. He then reads from a post he found on a recovery Facebook page with 1.5 million viewers: "But at some point some people are going to have to stand up for AA. Those people that judge us for protecting a program that has saved millions and millions of lives from those that would have their way of having people on narcotics sponsor others, be active members of AA, teaching people to be dependent upon God while they are actively dependent at best on a narcotic, well these people are not only dangerous to the very core of AA but they are also judgmental of AA and are sharing an opinion that is in direct conflict [with] our program." With almost biblical reverence for the AA literature, called "the Big Book," the Facebook post continues: "Your opinion almost killed you, try not to kill others with it. Call me a Big Book Thumper, an AA Nazi, whatever. I call you someone who is not in AA if you are against the Big Book and a detriment to others' sobriety. Once again, the Big Book is AA, your opinion is not."

3

THE PERILS AND PROMISES OF TREATMENT CENTERS

LISA'S SON, TOM, grew up in a supportive Northeastern middle-class family. As a result, Lisa does not understand why Tom experienced depression throughout his adolescence and young adulthood. Tom certainly had a better childhood than Lisa had had. True, he had witnessed his parents' divorce, but the divorce was relatively amicable, with both parents staying involved in his life.

Ironically, despite his history, Tom became a stand-up comedian. Work was stressful, though, and sometimes Tom didn't know when his next paycheck would arrive; other times, he was treated like a king by his fans and comedy club owners. Networking often included parties laden with drugs and alcohol, which is how Tom tried crack for the first time. Unfortunately, periodic crack use at parties escalated into regular crack use. Realizing he had a problem and having always had an open and honest relationship with Lisa, Tom finally told his mother that he needed help.

A self-described "mama bear," Lisa did everything she could to help Tom stop using crack. Lisa says, "I had to fight like mad to get him into treatment when he came to me and said he had become addicted to crack." Finally, Lisa got Tom into a residential treatment center after she spoke to "someone humane" at her insurance company. Treatment at the abstinence-only rehab center consisted of group counseling and twelve-step peer support groups. It did not include any kind of individualized mental health therapy for his depression, something that continues to upset Lisa even now because she is sure the depression contributed to his drug use. To make matters worse, the treatment center persuaded Tom to stop his antidepressant medication that had been prescribed by an outside psychiatrist. Then Tom met a friend at rehab who introduced him to heroin.

After leaving the treatment center, Tom began an almost daily quest for heroin, finding it even more addicting than crack. After a few months, Tom once again asked his mother for help. Fortunately, he was still on her health insurance—something hard to come by in the gig economy of stand-up comedy. Once again, he entered a rehab center. This abstinence-only treatment center consisted of detoxification, group counseling, and Alcoholics Anonymous: a combination for which insurance paid about $30,000 per month and Lisa paid coinsurance. After a month, the rehab center released Tom into a halfway house to live with other people in recovery and participate in AA meetings held on-site. Unfortunately for Tom and his family, this combination was not enough. Lisa says, "He was in twelve-step programs where people were very supportive of him, but it was unfortunately just a vicious cycle in which he would go into detox, then he would go into rehab, and he would go into holding. Then he would go into a halfway house and relapse. The halfway houses were usually just full of people using, and then it would start all over again. Or he would start to get well, and he would get a job, and once he had money, he would start to use again."

Then one day, Tom's grandmother saw a popular morning talk show on TV that described a fancy rehab center in California. Using an insurance broker, Lisa obtained a deal that seemed too good to be true: if she would just fly Tom out to California, insurance would pick up the whole tab for the ritzy rehab center, complete with a room for Tom on a bluff overlooking the ocean. Tom's sister called it Tom's "Make-A-Wish Foundation" gift. The rehab center included equine therapy, volleyball therapy, and a gym. It was the kind of place where movie stars went. They even involved the family in group therapy sessions, something relatively rare in Lisa's experience.

"[Tom] was a very earnest, patient participant in treatment," Lisa says. "When he was clean, he was so excited to be clean, and he had one hundred percent full participation. And all the counselors, when we had family time, just talked about how different he was and how he was going to make it."

As Tom's time in the luxury rehab came to an end, once more he faced having to endure the world outside the secure walls of residential treatment. But unlike the other rehab centers, this one gave him a parting gift: a shot of extended-release naltrexone, better known as Vivitrol.

"Totally life changing," Lisa says of the Vivitrol shot. "It eliminated not only his ability to get high with alcohol or any opioids, but his cravings were eliminated also."

Tom knew the shot really worked because after about one month, when the shot wore off, he started having drug-related dreams and terrible cravings. Unfortunately, the rehab center did not connect him to any long-term Vivitrol providers. The rehab center had emphasized that Vivitrol was not meant to be long-term treatment, just a jump start to recovery. Tom moved into a "sober home," just a more modern name for a halfway house, with other rehab graduates. But after two months of no rehab and no medication, he started using again. One day while high, he fell off a balcony and punctured his lung. Again, he contacted his mother. But this time Tom said he did not want a rehab center—he just wanted more of the medication that had worked for him.

Unfortunately, Tom had recently turned twenty-six years old and was no longer on his mother's health insurance. He had no stable job. He decided to move in with his grandmother in Oklahoma while he got his life back together. It would be a fresh start—Tom didn't really know anyone in Oklahoma.

Once he settled in with his grandmother, he searched for an outpatient provider of Vivitrol. He only found one provider in his city: a physician who offered both Suboxone and Vivitrol. But while the Suboxone was expensive for someone without insurance, the Vivitrol cost was impossible: over $1,000 per month.

Knowing Tom's financial and insurance situation, the physician strongly recommended Suboxone instead of Vivitrol, but according to Lisa, she and her entire family felt very judgmental about Suboxone: "It seemed like a terrible choice." All the rehab centers Tom had attended had spread the message to clients and families that Suboxone and methadone were widely misused and paths to another addiction. Lisa remembers eagerly awaiting Tom's phone call the day of his doctor's appointment, hoping for some good news, only to hear him say that he could afford the Suboxone but not the Vivitrol. Lisa remained silent on the other end of the line, which she thinks probably came off as disapproval of Suboxone. Tom left the clinic without a prescription for either medication. He was found dead from a heroin overdose a few days later.

IS IT POSSIBLE THAT TOM would have overdosed the next day or shortly thereafter even if he had received medication-assisted treatment? Anything is possible, but statistically, people on MAT, especially people treated with methadone or buprenorphine, have a far lower chance of dying from an opioid overdose than those without medication.[121,129,145–148] Vivitrol has not been studied nearly as extensively as Suboxone and other forms of oral buprenorphine, in part because Vivitrol has only been around for a few years. It also requires complete detoxification, which can be a significant hurdle for patients. Therefore, according to physicians I have interviewed, people who do well on it tend to have high levels of motivation, are white-collar professionals prohibited from using agonist treatments (i.e., methadone or buprenorphine) by their licenses, or are recently incarcerated individuals, meaning they have already been forced to undergo detoxification in jail or prison. Nevertheless, many people whom I have interviewed swear that Vivitrol has helped them with cravings and prevented them from getting high. In fact, the number one complaint about Vivitrol I hear from patients and family members is limited access—a reflection of few Vivitrol providers, exorbitant cost, and limited insurance coverage. And a growing body of research suggests that if you can overcome the detoxification, cost, and motivation barriers to start and continue extended-release naltrexone (big "ifs"), then the medication may be as effective as buprenorphine at preventing relapse.[59]

ADDICTION TREATMENT CENTERS can be characterized as residential or outpatient. Unlike standalone physicians who prescribe MAT to some patients while treating others for a wide range of health problems, addiction treatment centers focus on treating addiction, typically using a combination of counseling and peer support group methods. They often have an interdisciplinary team of providers, including counselors, social workers, and physicians. Given their specialization, these treatment centers may seem like an ideal place for people beginning recovery. But they are by no means easy to access and they do not necessarily provide evidence-based treatment options. During interviews with patients and family members, I am endlessly amazed by the number of "bad" treatment centers people go through before they find a "good" one.

Ian, who lives in a large Midwestern city, tried to enter a substance use disorder (SUD) treatment center multiple times, only to be put on a wait list. Finally, one of his friends suggested a tried-and-true method to getting in: "Call the hospital and say you are trying to kill yourself." Under federal law, hospitals are required to stabilize suicidal patients. According to Ian, when the emergency department physicians in his city realize the reason for the purported suicide attempt is drug addiction, they will push you to the front of the waiting line at local treatment centers. Ian has tried this method multiple times. He does not mention the fact that by getting to the front of the line he is pushing someone else further back. Nevertheless, immediate access to addiction treatment is critical. As Katie, an interviewee in recovery, explained, "It is the most crushing feeling when you finally reach out to get help and are turned away." That feeling can easily lead to relapse.

And once someone gets into an addiction treatment center, they are likely to be offered the same program, regardless of whether the place looks like a Four Seasons Hotel or a rundown mental health hospital: group counseling, Alcoholics Anonymous or Narcotics Anonymous, and wraparound nonmedical services to help people find jobs or housing. Sometimes education about the dangers of drugs is sprinkled in. Sometimes detoxification is part of the program, though often it is offered through a separate facility. Rarely are clients offered buprenorphine or naltrexone; they are almost never offered methadone. In 2016, only 27 percent of public addiction treatment centers offered buprenorphine.[149] Even fewer, 21 percent, offered naltrexone.[149] These numbers represent significant growth over the last ten years but are still shockingly low, especially given the exorbitant cost of attending the treatment centers.

Not only do most addiction treatment centers fail to offer MAT, residential treatment centers, colloquially referred to as "rehab," often actively dissuade patients from accessing these medications. Multiple interviewees have described not even considering MAT because rehab center employees had repeatedly told them that MAT was "just another drug." In particular, counselors with a history of recovery themselves through twelve-step programs are particularly likely to distrust MAT.[118,150–153]

A 2012 nationally representative study found that 20 percent of SUD treatment counselors knew little about methadone or buprenorphine effectiveness.[154] Aside from lack of accurate information, counselors who attribute personal responsibility to addiction may also be more likely to object to medications, perhaps because they think MAT "too easy" a recovery process.[155]

Fortunately, counselor training in MAT is associated with more positive attitudes toward it, suggesting that more training opportunities are needed.[154] Additionally, as more counselors become exposed to treatment centers using MAT, counselor attitudes toward MAT may improve. Such exposure is important, because in 2012, fewer than 6 percent of SUD counselors nationally were employed in a treatment program that prescribed methadone, fewer than 30 percent were employed in a treatment program that prescribed buprenorphine, and more than 70 percent worked in a program that prescribed neither.[154]

Perhaps most surprisingly, SUD counselors and mental health counselors are treated very differently in state regulations, with significantly lower education and training requirements for SUD counselors. This disparity mistakenly suggests that SUD counselors are less important or professional than mental health counselors, even though SUD counselors are a critical part of the workforce. Given the high co-occurrence of substance use and mental health disorders, one would expect a counselor trained in substance use disorders to also have training in mental health disorders and vice versa. But historically, education and training for the two professions diverged, primarily due to the stigma of substance use disorder. As a result, the majority of health care providers in addiction treatment centers during the twentieth century were people in recovery who had themselves primarily gone through twelve-step programs without graduate-level training.[156] Addiction treatment centers developed the assumption that if you had completed a twelve-step program successfully, you were qualified as an addiction counselor.[156] In contrast, training in evidence-based methods began far earlier for mental health counselors, which is reflected in their generally higher education and training requirements under state laws today.[156,157]

Only in the last twenty years did more formal credentialing for SUD counselors proliferate, largely due to the demands of managed care organizations who were paying for addiction treatment.[158]

Even today, twice as many states require licenses or credentialing for mental health counselors as for SUD counselors.[157] And when states do require licenses or credentialing for SUD counselors, fewer than 50 percent require a graduate degree; yet, 98 percent of states require *at least* a master's degree for mental health counselors.[157] The content of education for mental health counselors is also more likely to include client screening and treatment methods.[157] The authors of one comparative study argue that SUD counselors are more likely than mental health counselors to receive training through an apprentice-like system than through formal education, but the authors caution that the apprenticeship primarily occurs with other SUD counselors who are relying on twelve-step approaches, only sometimes including other evidence-based methods.[157]

An unfortunate result of the disparity in training between mental health counselors and SUD counselors is the underuse of evidence-based treatment in many addiction treatment centers.[157] Some scholars attribute this fact to difficulty of SUD counselors and addiction treatment center administrators in reading peer-reviewed literature, where evidence-based treatment is described.[157,159] Though almost two decades old now, a 2003 study in Wisconsin found that SUD counselors considered lack of time and difficulty reading peer-reviewed literature to be the top two barriers to evidence-based treatment adoption in their treatment centers.[159] Not surprisingly, it is easier to digest the information in peer-reviewed literature if you have been trained to do so in a graduate educational program.

Perhaps a better approach than the present laissez-faire attitude toward SUD counselor training would be for states to have equally high standards for SUD and mental health counselors, especially given the significant overlap in populations with SUD and mental health disorders. At the same time, states could bolster funding for peer support specialists who do not need advanced educational training but provide critical support and inspiration based on their personal recovery stories. Those peer support specialists who also want to provide counseling could become SUD counselors by meeting state counseling education/training requirements.

Ideally, SUD treatment centers that receive state or federal funding would be required to employ a mixture of both types of professionals: SUD counselors with formal evidence-based treatment training and peer support counselors with lived recovery experience. As one SUD client told me, "You need a mixture of architects and builders," meaning people who are formally trained in building and people who have actual experience laying stone. One scholar writes, "At face value, it appears that mental health counselors are closer to being able to address dual diagnoses than are drug abuse counselors."[157] To bring the existing SUD counselor workforce up to date, their employers, namely treatment centers, will need to give them time and funding for education.

GROUP COUNSELING is the most common treatment method available in both residential treatment centers and intensive outpatient programs (IOPs). IOPs are an alternative to rehab—allowing patients to continue living at home and working or going to school while attending treatment multiple times per week on an outpatient basis, for hours at a time. While group counseling forms the backbone of rehab and IOPs, individual counseling is far rarer. Even though some reviews suggest that individual counseling and group counseling may be equally effective for addiction, there are some strong caveats to these reviews. First, most clinical trials of addiction counseling have looked at individual counseling, not group counseling, probably because the latter is harder to study.[160] Second, in practice, group counseling has been poorly defined, with vast potential differences in how it is provided from treatment center to treatment center. Therefore, while group counseling with evidence-based components, such as motivational interviewing, may be effective, other types of group counseling, such as those focused on the facilitator educating the clients, have essentially no evidence base.[160] According to a recent study, "Remarkably little research exists concerning what substance use disorder clinicians do in group therapy."[160]

When clients choose a treatment center, they are unlikely to know whether they are getting effective or ineffective group counseling. In residential treatment, they are unlikely to know the nature or purpose of the group until they have enrolled in the program and moved in. In most cases, there will be a preset list and order of groups that clients must attend with little ability to choose between them.

Interviewees have described a wide spectrum of group counseling experiences, from very positive to very negative. Even the purpose and structure of the groups can differ widely from treatment center to treatment center. For example, some groups are led by a recent college graduate without a therapy license or addiction experience who reads straight from a workbook, with limited participant engagement. One interviewee likens this to "adult daycare." Other groups are led by an individual experienced in recovery or a licensed therapist, with participants prompted to share and respond to others' experiences. Some groups are very structured, while others are free-flowing. Some groups focus entirely on facilitating participation in the twelve steps, while other groups have nothing to do with the twelve steps, focusing instead on relapse prevention or drug education.

It is much easier for a treatment center to offer group counseling than individual therapy, especially evidence-based individual therapy. Unlike individual therapy, which typically requires a licensed clinical professional with a Master of Social Work or a PhD in psychology, group counseling does not necessarily require these credentials. For example, a bachelor's degree or even a high school degree with an online counseling certification is typically sufficient for a group focused on educating clients about the dangers of drug use or facilitating participation in the twelve steps. Therefore, it is easier to hire staff to lead group counseling. Furthermore, group counseling is obviously more cost effective for treatment centers as more clients can participate in it at any given time. In the vast majority of cases, when new clients or patients arrive at the treatment center, they are simply added to an existing counseling group with open spots, a process called open enrolling, regardless of the potential mismatch between participants.[160] It is no wonder that group counseling is the norm, especially when revenue is tight.

In her book *Inside Rehab: The Surprising Truth about Addiction Treatment—and How to Get Help That Works*, Anne Fletcher describes traveling to numerous residential rehab centers in which she sees the same pattern: group counseling combined with twelve-step support. In my own research, I have found the same regimen. And while interviewees routinely proclaim the benefits of individual therapy, they are often on the fence about group counseling. Considering the strong association between trauma, mental health disorders, and addiction, I am not surprised that some interviewees explicitly prefer individual counseling over group counseling. I ask Lisa, Tom's mother, to describe based on her son's experience what a good rehab center should provide. She says, "More individual counseling . . . the thirty-thousand-a-month treatment wasn't more helpful because people were treated like spa patients; it was more effective because it offered individual counseling and medical treatment. And so, what would be needed is decent pay for social workers so that you could have a consistent, professional staff providing individual therapy to help people understand why they're destroying their own lives."

In contrast, group counseling is much more difficult to individualize. Interviewees have described being thrown into groups where they are forced to listen to someone else's problems with minimal one-to-one counselor interaction, sometimes resulting in an entire session wherein only a few individuals' problems were addressed. I often hear interviewees say that group counseling should at least include people in the same stage of recovery or with the same types of mental health issues, rather than a potpourri of people with different health problems. For example, Alice in Indiana believes she has benefited from group counseling at the Veterans Health Administration for women with a history of sexual assault, but she says she would stop talking if a man were to join the group. Jake, who is in recovery and has worked as a counselor in many Florida rehab centers, says he frequently sees men and women mixed together in groups, where the women stop talking altogether. Similarly, interviewees criticize the notion of people with very different SUD problems being lumped together in one group. Describing her son's participation in an IOP in a Midwestern state, Rachel says, "Everyone [was grouped together]. From one guy because he got caught with one joint—one little joint—to one guy who was shooting up heroin four times a day, every day . . . no one could relate to anybody."

The relative underuse of individual counseling points to a systemic problem in rehab centers and IOPs: lack of treatment individualization. Lack of individualization is related to an even broader problem in treatment centers: lack of person-centered care. Person-centered care essentially means health care where the patient is the CEO of his or her own journey. It includes shared decision-making and patient choice in treatment. It means letting patients pick their own goals and helping them make a treatment plan accordingly. In contrast, patients in rehab centers and IOPs typically receive a cookie-cutter approach to treatment with only some limited choices.

One component of "one size fits all" is mandatory twelve-step participation, whether or not the individual wants it and even though forcing a spiritual support group onto someone who is uncomfortable with spirituality is inappropriate. Sometimes the spirituality morphs into religiosity. Lisa says, "My son really struggled with his faith, his lack of belief in God . . . it couldn't help but rub him the wrong way when he had counselors say, 'You're really never going to get better until you accept Jesus into your heart.' I mean, things like that are just not appropriate. People's faith should not be held over them." Even though Tom never attended a rehab center that advertised itself as spiritual or religious, such mandates crept in. To this day, Lisa does not understand why prayer was supposed to be an answer to her son's deadly medical condition.

Even some AA adherents think it's a scam to pay for treatment centers focused on AA meetings, which are already freely available in the community. According to Jessica, who is in recovery, "You can pay fifty thousand dollars to go to treatment and they sit you down and it's an AA service. If I'm going to pay a few thousand dollars, I want some intensive therapy. I want my own therapy."

Treatment center providers and administrators say they must introduce clients to twelve-step meetings in their residential facility if clients are eventually going to participate in twelve-step meetings outside of the facility. Treatment centers often view twelve-step meetings in the community as aftercare; so, they are essentially preparing clients to transition into what will become their long-term recovery method. This is a valid argument if clients want to participate in twelve-steps groups during and after residential treatment. But if that's all the treatment center is doing, with some twelve-step-focused group counseling thrown in, then clients and their families are being underserved at great expense. After all, clients typically have at least a month in a residential facility to focus on their recovery without the distractions of work and family, meaning there is plenty of time for regular individualized therapy.

Kyle, another counselor in recovery himself, sums up the one-size-fits-all problem as follows: "The goal if you go to treatment or seek treatment is to complete the program with abstinence and not come up positive on a urine analysis. It's just a really ineffective system and it's all based on this twelve-step modality that has kind of been allowed to run unchecked. It's really hard to do research on it. There's no way to really tell if it's effective or not."

He's right, it is very difficult to research treatment center efficacy. For example, residential treatment centers are rarely required to report long-term results to authorities. Instead, if they are even required to report any results, they report urine drug screens of people currently enclosed within the rehab center—a time when even the least evidence-based centers can expect negative urine drug screens, so long as the rehab center has a good security system. Repeatedly, interviewees describe "doing great" in rehab, only to relapse the day after leaving. Instead, rehab centers should report results collected months or even years later. Furthermore, results should not be limited to urine drug screen analyses. They should include broader quality of life indicators, including whether the patient has a job, housing, and a regular physician; is staying out of the criminal justice system; and has met his or her own goals. Fortunately, treatment centers that receive federal substance abuse block grants from the Substance Abuse and Mental Health Services Administration must include many of these broader measures in their reporting requirements,[161] but such block grants only account for 16 percent of total SUD public financing in the United States. Many one-size-fits-all treatment centers that rely on private money or commercial insurance miss out on these important quality indicators, focusing more on short-term urine drug screens, which incidentally is big business for rehabs, with comedian John Oliver calling urine in rehab "liquid gold."

Most states require licensure or certification of addiction treatment centers, regardless of whether the center receives government funding. However, licensure or certification requirements vary widely from state to state and can be pretty limited. For example, according to a 2013 study, only about half of states set standards for a program director. Rarely is such a program director required to have a medical degree, except when the program provides methadone treatment or is hospital-based. About half of states set standards regarding counselor to client ratios, and counselor education and training requirements vary significantly from state to state. Additionally, even though almost all states require creation of a treatment plan at the time of client entry, only ten states require aftercare or follow-up services for clients leaving treatment. Shockingly, in twenty-six states there are no data reporting requirements for licensure.[162]

I routinely ask interviewees what makes a good treatment center. One of the most common responses is a center wherein clients choose their own treatment modalities from a wide variety of available methods. "You should offer everything," Kyle says. "A good facility should be able to handle anything within the vein of drug and alcohol use or abuse. If you can only handle a forty-five-year-old alcoholic who's willing to engage in the twelve steps and practice spirituality, then you're not a substance abuse treatment center, you're this specific consumer treatment facility. And that's fine, that's okay if you recognize the limits of your professional ability and you say this is where I'm effective. But that needs to be communicated to everybody." In other words, some people may genuinely want a standard abstinence-only treatment program, but they should know up front that's what they are getting and that there are other effective options from which to choose.

Explaining an ideal hypothetical treatment center, Doug, who has been through rehab multiple times, suggests that treatment centers offer services in the framework of the biopsychosocial model of addiction. He would offer MAT to address the physiological components of addiction; evidence-based counseling and mental health medication to address the psychological and mental health components; peer support groups to address the spiritual components; and educational, employment, and housing services to address the social components. Even if a treatment center lacks the staff or resources to provide all of these services, it should at least connect patients to outside providers who can fill in the gaps. The key word here though is "offer," not "force."

Almost no interviewees described attending residential and outpatient treatment centers with client-directed treatment choices. Mandy, a parent trying to navigate the Midwestern addiction treatment landscape with her son, was one of the few. She described the best residential program attended by him, where on the first day administrators asked, "Do you want to be in a twelve-step program?"

and her son responded, "I've done so much of that now . . . I think traditional counseling is what I need. I think I need to get to the base of why I made these decisions in the first place." The treatment center then let him skip the twelve-step support groups and beefed up the schedule with individual counseling sessions.

Even fewer treatment centers approach addiction treatment through a harm reduction lens, which Stan believes means helping patients meet their own goals, regardless of whether that goal is complete abstinence from drug use. He says, "Honestly, I would just want to meet every single patient where they're at, whether they're still sticking a needle in their arm or not, whether they want to be completely abstinent or not, whether they want to be on MAT or not, wherever that individual wants to be, I want to have a resource for them."

My favorite description of an ideal treatment center comes from Tyrese, who recovered from opioid addiction with the help of both buprenorphine and twelve-step support groups. He describes a "pick your own path" approach to treatment center design, like picking a college major, where patients can select a religious track, twelve-step track, MAT track, counseling track, or some combination. "And if, God forbid, you come back as a repeat, obviously something didn't work, you can either go back through and see what may have not worked in the path that you already did and redo that path, or you can change the path and find your solution. Because everyone's different." Unfortunately, he has never witnessed this treatment design, despite being in and out of treatment centers for a decade.

Person-centered care also means recognizing that addiction is a relapsing, chronic condition. Over time, effective treatment will lead to fewer relapses, and hopefully eventually to no relapses. But residential treatment centers have traditionally approached addiction as an acute short-term condition for which a quick thirty-day stint is a cure. The short-term perspective prevents adequate care transition from residential to outpatient settings. Similarly, a short-term perspective prevents rehab centers that start MAT from explaining to patients that they may need to be on MAT for a long time, like in Tom's case. Not surprisingly, rehab centers often treat relapse with another stint in the same rehab center using the same program rather than recommending an alternate program. In the meantime, family members find themselves digging into retirement savings yet again.

Many readers may be shocked to learn that not everyone needs a residential treatment setting to begin with. It seems that anytime someone in a movie or TV show has a drug problem, they are sent to residential rehab. Yet studies suggest that IOPs are just as effective as residential treatment, and evidence for residential treatment efficacy is mixed.[163,164]

As one well-respected addiction psychiatrist explained to me, the people most likely to benefit from a residential setting have severe co-occurring disorders, are pregnant, or need to separate themselves from their home environment, such as when family members are using drugs. But not everyone falls into these categories. An individual with a strong and stable support network who lacks a severe co-occurring disorder may do better in an IOP than residential treatment, because the IOP would allow him or her to continue work, attend school, and have regular interactions with family. For some people, work, school, and family are their motivations for recovery, so taking away these motivations can be harmful.

Even one month away from college classes to participate in rehab rather than an IOP, for example, could cause a student to fall significantly behind in her studies, marring her self-esteem or decreasing her motivation to graduate. Additionally, not everyone has the luxury of being able to take time off work to go to a rehab center for a month or more. The United States has limited legal protection for people who take time away from work to focus on their health. The federal Family and Medical Leave Act requires employers to hold a position open for someone facing a health crisis or to provide a substantially similar position after twelve weeks, but the law only applies if the employer has at least fifty employees and if the employee has worked there full-time for at least one year. So, restaurant servers, people in the gig economy, people who work in small businesses, and many others are out of luck. Even when the law applies, the person will be unpaid during the twelve-week period, something family breadwinners can scarcely afford.

And relative to IOPs, people in residential settings may feel more trapped or coerced into the treatment methods provided, with limited outside communication. Many interviewees have described jail-like settings in residential treatment, with phone calls to family or significant others being highly restricted, non-twelve-step reading material being forbidden, and internet-enabled devices being confiscated.

Not only should relapse be expected during addiction treatment, but patients should be accepted with open arms by providers when they do relapse. Instead, many treatment centers kick patients out if they have a positive urine drug screen. Unfortunately, even outpatient treatment centers that provide MAT frequently "fire" patients if they misuse a drug—even marijuana. Alternatively, some treatment centers refuse to provide MAT until an individual has eliminated all forms of drug use, except opioids. Other treatment centers refuse to provide MAT until an individual has successfully completed counseling first. Frustrated, Elise, who is in recovery, told me, "Addiction is the only disease where you have to get better in order to get treated."

Such treatment centers are referred to as "high barrier" or "high threshold" treatment centers. In contrast, "low barrier" treatment centers accept all patients, even providing MAT to patients who are still misusing other drugs or who are sometimes skipping their medication and misusing opioids. Low-barrier treatment centers lack zero-tolerance policies and lack counseling or other adjunctive treatment requirements, though they often recommend counseling and peer support groups to clients. Low-barrier treatment centers do not have predetermined medication dosages, MAT time limits, or cookie-cutter treatment programs for each patient. Instead, the providers work with the patient to meet his or her goals, continuing medication if the patient feels that the medication is helping, even if relapse still sometimes occurs or other drugs are misused.

We often address other diseases with a low-barrier approach. For example, we do not cancel patients' bipolar disorder or depression prescriptions just because they sometimes skip doses or do not use the medication exactly as prescribed. As a society, we take the pragmatic approach of acknowledging that it is better to guide the patient back into a regular medication routine than to leave the patient without effective treatment. And considering how difficult it is for people to join addiction treatment centers to begin with, kicking them out may spell the end of treatment altogether. Yet in addiction treatment, a punitive approach still often predominates, wherein if you don't take your MAT as prescribed or as often as prescribed, then you will never get it again.

Not only is low-barrier MAT treatment more pragmatic than high-barrier treatment, an increasing body of evidence suggests that it is more effective at retaining patients in buprenorphine treatment,[165] and retention in buprenorphine treatment is associated with a dramatic drop in overdose mortality.[14] Additionally, researchers are on the fence about whether counseling should be added to office-based buprenorphine treatment, with a recent systematic review finding that half of the studies saw a positive effect from adding counseling and half of the studies saw no effect from adding counseling.[166] Counseling can be a great addition if the patient wants it, but we should not discourage people from taking potentially lifesaving medication simply because they do not want counseling. In 2019, in their consensus statement titled *Medications for Opioid Use Disorder Save Lives*, the National Academies of Sciences, Engineering, and Medicine explicitly stated that withholding MAT for any reason, including for lack of participation in behavioral treatments, is unjust and unethical.[28]

Having come to the same realization, the Substance Abuse and

Mental Health Services Administration, a federal agency, is now encouraging providers to prescribe MAT without strings attached, including without counseling if patients are uninterested in counseling.[23] Such an approach wildly differs from what I have observed in many treatment centers across the United States. The protocol also encourages providers to prescribe MAT even if patients are still misusing opioids and other drugs, including benzodiazepines, because on balance MAT is likely to lead to decreased opioid misuse and lower overdose risks.

The government's advice reflects common sense. As numerous interviewees have told me, if you kick someone out of a treatment center or take away their medication, they will almost certainly relapse. If anything, relapse is a sign that more intensive treatment is needed, such as greater counseling frequency or a higher medication dose. Unfortunately, as hard as it is to find an addiction treatment center accepting new patients, it can be even harder to find a treatment center that will accept you and provide MAT with no strings attached. In fact, I didn't see such treatment centers firsthand until I visited the very progressive state of Washington.

RECOVERY WORKS (not its real name) is a multilevel treatment center that treats a wide range of substance use disorders, but it is their approach to opioid addiction treatment that I am most interested in. The three-story building is nestled among middle-class residences at the edge of a metropolis. When you enter the building, it doesn't look special; you see aqua-colored walls, a receptionist area, and a waiting room with a stack of NA brochures. A sign on the wall lists patients' rights and a flyer describes weekly job training opportunities with the local food industry. Perhaps the most unusual sight, though, is a stack of brochures that describe the benefits of carrying the opioid antidote naloxone (also known by the brand name Narcan), something many treatment centers refuse to discuss lest they imply the very realistic possibility that patients may relapse.

Near the front entrance lies a family visitation room, where I conduct my interviews. Other than a few chairs and a window, the family visitation room is empty. It is certainly not the luxurious, spa-like atmosphere of the California rehab attended by Tom. Practically all of Recovery Works' patients are on Medicaid, and Medicaid programs don't usually pay for unnecessary, unproven frills.

The basement of the facility houses a detoxification center where patients might stay for a few days. After detoxification, patients can choose to move upstairs to the residential treatment area where they stay up to a month, or they can be immediately connected to affiliated outpatient providers. The upstairs residential treatment facility holds approximately fifteen beds due to a former Medicaid rule preventing payment for more beds, presumably to encourage shifting patients to outpatient treatment. Also upstairs, patients get group counseling, individual therapy, drug education, and if they so choose, twelve-step support groups. But the program is not twelve-step-based. Group counseling focuses on cognitive behavioral therapy skills and coping skills rather than twelve-step facilitation. Uniquely, patients are also invited to participate in a harm reduction group, where they discuss how to prevent overdose in the event of relapse, including carrying naloxone and snorting rather than injecting drugs, thereby lowering the drugs' bioavailability.

The residential treatment center is beginning to provide MAT to eligible patients who want it, but providers have faced serious practical hurdles. For example, since no pharmacy exists on site and too few local physicians and nurses are willing to work in rehab centers, storing and administering buprenorphine by staff initially proved difficult. To manage daily oral buprenorphine administration, the treatment center installed a buprenorphine "vending machine." Approved staff can access the machine, which tracks dispensing for purposes of Medicaid reimbursement. Methadone is currently unavailable, because logistically it would be nearly impossible to transport patients to the local methadone clinic daily from the residential treatment center. According to the staff, extended-release naltrexone is the easiest to store and administer, given that any nurse can mix and inject the medication, which is not a controlled substance.

Even though the residential facility is relatively unique in providing MAT, not all the staff are on board. As Dana, a nurse, describes, "Some of the counselors are in recovery themselves and they don't feel comfortable even being opioid adjacent. Even giving [Suboxone] to someone and seeing them take it can be tough for the counselors themselves." Importantly, Recovery Works recognizes that some patients do not want MAT: "Just because we embrace harm reduction doesn't mean we exclude abstinence." In other words, patients get choices in their care.

When patients complete residential treatment at Recovery Works, they leave with a carefully drafted, mutually agreed upon transition plan to outpatient treatment. The transition is seamless, too, given that Recovery Works is a network with multiple outpatient treatment facilities to which patients are directly connected. Medical records and insurance information follow the patient. Some of the residential treatment providers even work in the outpatient treatment facility part-time, further ensuring continuity of care.

Most of Recovery Works' patients are outpatient. They do not typically go through the residential treatment facility, although some patients do complete detoxification at the residential facility prior to beginning outpatient treatment. I ask the medical director, an addiction psychiatrist, to categorize which patients are most likely to benefit from residential treatment prior to outpatient treatment. She responds, "I think those who would score as having a more severe use disorder. People with polysubstance use, long-term use, IV use versus smoking, unstable housing, or just a very chaotic social situation. I think simply having a place to rest for a while, that in and of itself would be very helpful for them." In contrast, she describes patients for whom outpatient treatment is probably sufficient as "the white-collar opioid use disorder folks who still maintain a good job, and they have a family, and they've been using pills, [snorting] them, and have lots of underlying structure in place that's going to help with their recovery." Even though these general categories may not apply to all patients, they do indicate the extent to which patient characteristics are considered in an individualized decision-making process. Client participation for thirty days in residential treatment is significantly more lucrative for a treatment center than thirty days in outpatient treatment, so the medical director's attitude indicates a decision-making process in which dollars are not the priority.

Although incorporating MAT into the Recovery Works residential treatment center has been difficult logistically, Dana believes that residential treatment centers in general are a golden opportunity to introduce people to MAT if they want it. She says, "If you have OUD [opioid use disorder], sometimes it's hard to adhere to your medication. In a controlled environment [such as a residential treatment center], it's being given to you every day at a structured time, and it's really being treated as a medication. I think that really locks in the idea that this is treatment. This is a medication. You take it every day at the same time rather than in response to either withdrawal symptoms or situational triggers, if that makes sense. That's something I've really been coaching people on. Behaviorally, this medication's going to be much more effective if you take it as a medication." Dana is referring to the fact that many patients at Recovery Works have previously tried buprenorphine on the streets to prevent withdrawal symptoms at random times, but they have not taken it regularly to treat the addiction. Without taking it at regular times as prescribed, people do not experience the full benefit of the medication, especially the physiological stability it enables.

In addition to the Recovery Works residential facility working closely with its outpatient facility, the outpatient treatment facility is low-barrier and operates on a "hub-and-spoke" model. Patients seeking buprenorphine or extended-release naltrexone treatment first go to the outpatient hub, where they begin treatment within a few days—a rarity in much of the United States. Once stabilized in the hub, patients are moved to the spokes, meaning other affiliated outpatient providers, with whom patients can continue treatment long term. This version of the hub-and-spoke model, which exists in various forms throughout the country, allows many patients to access MAT quickly despite the existence of federally imposed patient limits for buprenorphine. In fact, the Recovery Works outpatient hub never quite reaches maximum patient capacity despite large patient demand because transfer to the spokes occurs regularly. If patients want abstinence-only treatment, then the hub will connect them to relevant, non-MAT-providing spokes.

I visited the Recovery Works outpatient hub, about a fifteen-minute drive from the residential treatment center. Even though it's located in a low-income area with recent African immigrants trying to make ends meet, the building looks new and inviting from the outside with well-maintained landscaping. The waiting room is more pleasant than that of the residential treatment facility. It has a play area for children, lots of magazines for reading, inspirational posters on the wall, potted plants, and plenty of light shining through windows. Basically, it is a well-run facility that makes patients feel like they are in a regular physician's office—and they are.

The hub utilizes a low-barrier, harm reduction approach to oral buprenorphine treatment. Extended-release naltrexone is also available but rarely requested by patients. Most patients desiring buprenorphine will receive the medication quickly. There are no strings attached. Patients often participate in counseling on site or at associated counselors' offices since counseling is always encouraged but never required. Nor is participation in peer support groups required, though plenty of support group brochures stand on end tables in the lobby. Urine drug screens occur regularly, not as a punitive mechanism to catch "bad" patients, but rather as a treatment tool to help providers decide appropriate dosages or medication adjustments if the current treatment approach doesn't seem to be working.

Patients are provided resources for recovering from other disorders, such as cocaine use disorder, but patients are never kicked out of the program for using other drugs. According to the staff, if patients were to be kicked out for misusing other drugs, they would simply continue using those drugs *plus* they would return to misusing opioids—a fact consistently confirmed by interviewees in recovery. Surely misuse of one drug is better than misuse of two. Providers critically observe possible interactions between buprenorphine and concomitant benzodiazepine misuse, a potentially dangerous combination, but they do not automatically cease the opioid addiction treatment.

Even if buprenorphine is not consistently found in the patient's urine drug screens, indicating that patients are missing or selling some doses, providers are pleased if buprenorphine is usually present. Regular buprenorphine treatment with periodic stopping followed by periodic heroin misuse is considered better than regular heroin misuse. If patients are suspected of selling their buprenorphine because it is not appearing in the urine drug screens, providers try to assess why the patient is diverting it. Often the reason is as simple as helping a significant other or friend prevent withdrawal symptoms, in which case the provider recommends introducing that person to formal treatment at the hub. Dana says such introductions are important because many people purchasing buprenorphine on the street don't frame the medication as potential treatment or don't understand addiction as a medical condition, rather they simply view buprenorphine as "that thing that stops me from feeling sick."

Importantly, hub staff consciously try to implement person-centered care. They use motivational interviewing, following patients' leads in treatment rather than trying to impose a predetermined treatment plan. Dana, who works at both the outpatient hub and the residential center, says, "We're going to walk alongside you during your recovery path, but you decide where that path goes. We're not going to put a leash on you and drag you along the path that we choose."

I ask how the hub is perceived in the community, especially by local politicians. Does the public health department support it? Dana responds, "Oh, definitely." The main point person in the public health department is not only a big fan of harm reduction in general but he even supports supervised consumption sites. The Recovery Works network gets funding and technical support from the public health department, which also helps the network navigate the Medicaid bureaucracy.

Despite the paperwork involved in accepting Medicaid patients, Dana is very proud of the fact that Washington's Medicaid program covers 100 percent of the costs associated with oral buprenorphine and extended-release naltrexone treatment, including detoxification if needed prior to medication induction, ongoing physician appointments, adjunctive counseling, and of course, the prescriptions themselves. Furthermore, no prior authorization is required for sublingual buprenorphine up to 24 mg (a higher than average dose) or for extended-release naltrexone. Providers in other states face far greater MAT barriers from their Medicaid programs, especially in the form of prior authorization requirements or limited detoxification coverage. In fact, Dana says that patients in Washington have better Medicaid coverage than private insurance coverage for MAT, a sentiment I have never heard expressed in any other state.

AFTER VISITING RECOVERY WORKS, I took a cab to the lowest-barrier treatment center I have ever seen. I had to reread the instructions to confirm that the treatment center was indeed located in a Methodist church. Once I arrived at the church, I was told to take the stairs to a basement where I would find a range of recovery and social support services, including buprenorphine treatment.

If the church's mission is to reach the homeless and outcast, then it has clearly succeeded. Homeless people and their few, meager possessions line the streets. A few thrift stores, bars, and local coffee shops are the only signs of local industry. As instructed, I reach the church basement, and I encounter a long hallway with many doors. In one room is the syringe exchange program and in another a naloxone distribution center. Further down the hall is a temporary shelter for homeless adolescents. Through a fourth door are basic supplies for surviving the outdoors, ranging from blankets to sleeping bags. Finally, a nondescript door opens into a nurse practitioner's office.

The walls of the office are covered in colorful framed artwork, giving you the feeling of walking into a rainbow. On one side is a patient examination table; on the other side are a large desk, bookshelves, and potted plants. A petite, soft-spoken blonde woman in her midfifties introduces herself as the nurse practitioner. This room in the church basement is the hub of a neighborhood hub-and-spoke system (unrelated to Recovery Works). The basement room is also a place where people walking in from the street can obtain HIV and hepatitis C testing on demand, followed by referrals to treatment and Medicaid.

I ask the nurse practitioner how she handles her responsibilities despite only being able to prescribe buprenorphine to up to thirty patients at once, since nurse practitioners currently have tighter buprenorphine patient limits than physicians, who can have more than thirty patients after one year of having a SAMHSA waiver. Surely, she is bursting at the seams with patients. She smiles coyly and explains that that problem has been solved by quickly connecting patients to spokes in the community—particularly a chain of private psychiatric clinics with whom she has a close relationship. When those clinics reach their own patient limits, she connects patients to other potential spokes—though that can be difficult when other physicians sometimes do not adopt her low-barrier, harm reduction philosophy. If providers don't follow a harm reduction philosophy, they sometimes prematurely discharge patients, eventually returning them to her hub only to be reconnected with another spoke later.

The nurse practitioner is operating on a shoestring budget but says she loves every minute of her work, which includes seeing changes in the local, vulnerable population who sometimes become sufficiently stabilized to exit homelessness. At the very least, they finally receive care for related, debilitating conditions, such as HIV.

Before I can ask more questions, she abruptly ends our interview. A homeless individual is approaching her office, asking if this is where he can get addiction treatment. She welcomes him inside, shutting the door in front of me. She has more important work to do.

4

METHADONE CLINICS

Maintaining Stigma for Decades

MELISSA WAS FIGHTING her abusive ex-husband for custody of their young son amid a three-year-long divorce process. Her mother had recently passed away, leaving Melissa without family support. A licensed practical nurse in the local hospital, she struggled to care for patients as her own life disintegrated—not that her life had ever been easy.

As a young child, Melissa had survived a traumatic car accident, one in which she witnessed her uncle, the driver, die. For years she received regular steroid injections for the resulting chronic back pain. Back then physicians never offered her opioid treatment, except for the few days in the hospital immediately following the accident. But times were different now. In the hospital, Melissa saw physicians routinely prescribing opioids for chronic pain. Nevertheless, she had never seriously considered opioids as a treatment option for her back pain until Elizabeth, an older nurse practitioner in the same hospital, offered Melissa some of her own Lortab, a brand name for the opioid hydrocodone.

Perhaps Elizabeth understood what she was doing—introducing a vulnerable single mother to a highly addictive narcotic. Or maybe Elizabeth truly thought Lortab would help manage Melissa's pain with few repercussions. Her exact words to Melissa had been, "I think this will help your back." Or maybe Elizabeth meant the Lortab to serve as a kind of antidepressant for her coworker, one who was clearly struggling to get through each twelve-hour shift. Either way, Elizabeth, who according to Melissa is "unfortunately no longer with us in body," eventually caught onto the fact that that her colleague had become fully addicted. Nevertheless, Elizabeth continued supplying Melissa with more and more pills. To Melissa, Lortabs were miracle pills, boosting her mood and energy while relieving her physical pain. Explaining her relationship with Elizabeth, Melissa said, "I think we saw each other eye to eye for what it was. I felt an underlying connection with her, like this is what it is and it's not ethical, but hey, we are working, we are helping people with serious illnesses in the hospital."

But soon the sporadic pills provided by Elizabeth were not enough, and Melissa went one step further—she called in a Lortab prescription to the Walmart pharmacy under Elizabeth's name. Elizabeth was, after all, a nurse practitioner who could prescribe opioids for patients. When no one noticed, Melissa did it again, soon establishing a routine. The state's prescription drug monitoring program was not yet mandatory or else pharmacists might have noticed, though Melissa believes she prompted the change in her state's prescription drug monitoring regulation. Not surprisingly, until then, physicians and nurses already pressed for time rarely checked the prescription drug monitoring program since they were not required to do so.

Then one day out of the blue, Melissa had a call from her friend, Ashley, another licensed practical nurse. Ashley collaborated with the state's nurse licensing board on investigating ethical violations, and Melissa's name had come up. Over the phone, Ashley warned Melissa: "Don't pick up any more prescriptions. If you do, the police will be waiting for you." Melissa didn't pick up her next Lortab prescription, but the licensing board still contacted her a few days later. They believed she was illicitly and fraudulently prescribing herself opioids. An ethics hearing would be held wherein the board would decide whether to suspend her nursing license.

Technically, Melissa could have brought an attorney to the hearing, but she couldn't afford one. And since it was an ethical violations case rather than a criminal case, the government had no obligation to provide her with an attorney. After exhaustively reviewing relevant prescription records, the board suspended Melissa's nursing license. They listed her name with her picture on the board's public website, humiliating her. Her ex-husband used this information to win sole custody of their child, claiming that it was in the best interests of the child to stay away from Melissa. To get her nursing license back, Melissa needed to attend an addiction treatment program for nurses followed by a probationary period of working under another nurse.

The mandatory abstinence-based treatment program prohibited medication-assisted treatment. The program emphasized twelve-step group attendance, something evidenced by a paper supposedly signed by the weekly Alcoholics Anonymous or Narcotics Anonymous chairperson. Of course, AA and NA are anonymous, so it is virtually impossible for authorities to ensure compliance, since they cannot obtain the chairperson's name or contact information, except for a scribbled signature. Melissa grudgingly attended a few AA meetings. She didn't see what God or spirituality had to do with her addiction. Plus, amid withdrawals and serious cravings, she didn't pay much attention to the discussions. So Melissa stopped going to AA, instead forging the rotating anonymous chairperson's signature on documents submitted to the licensing board.

In addition to twelve-step group attendance, the board required participation in group counseling sessions. These she likewise found ineffective as they basically repeated the information provided in AA by helping you "work through the steps" with worksheets and forced discussion. Despite having found the entire mandatory treatment process a joke, Melissa passed with flying colors, and the nursing board temporarily reinstated her under another nurse for a probationary period. But Melissa's physical and psychological cravings and emotional problems remained.

Shortly after beginning the probationary period in a different hospital unit, Melissa resumed her old game. Except this time, using a different nurse practitioner's information, Melissa called in prescriptions for a friend. The friend picked up the prescriptions and split the pills with Melissa. It wasn't too long before the nurse under whom Melissa worked noticed the classic signs of opioid use: pinpoint pupils, nodding off, and constant itching. Clearly, Melissa was misusing again. But the supervising nurse had no proof of actual misuse or diversion, so she didn't report it. Perhaps it was nurse camaraderie, an instinct to protect each other against intrusive authority. Nevertheless, the supervising nurse fired Melissa for nebulous reasons, likely to protect herself from any potential liability.

Jobless and childless, Melissa felt hopeless and worthless. She had tried multiple times to quit cold turkey, but it had never worked. As a last resort, she drove to the closest methadone clinic, about one hour away. She felt strangely out of place there despite being surrounded by people with the same problem: compulsive opioid misuse despite terrible consequences. Perhaps it was the part of town in which the clinic was located, with homeless people and empty beer cans lining the sidewalk, only a liquor store and some gas stations in sight, that made her feel so uncomfortable. But with nothing left to lose, Melissa walked into the methadone clinic, briefly explained her situation to the receptionist, and was told to return in five days.

A few days later, Melissa drove the hour-long distance to the methadone clinic. It was strangely empty this time, since her appointment took place during nondosing hours. The physician examined her, asked for a urine sample, and took a full history. Melissa held nothing back. He prescribed the minimum methadone dose and told her to return for her medication the next day at 5:00 a.m. Technically, she could come any time between 5:00 and 7:00 a.m., but people with jobs, disabilities, or young kids got priority, and the line could be very long. Melissa was advised to come early. She then briefly met with a counselor who gave her a mental health history assessment to determine any additional psychological needs.

The next day, Melissa began a two-year routine of waking up at 3:00 a.m., dressing, eating breakfast, and driving the hour to the methadone clinic. By 4:00 a.m., cars and people on foot circled the block, waiting for the clinic to open. At 5:00 a.m., the doors opened. Patients would check in with a receptionist, who seemed to always be counting piles of cash since the clinic did not accept Medicaid and few patients had commercial insurance. After paying, patients lined up as if waiting for a popular Disney ride. Once Melissa finally got to the front of the line, a technician directed her to one of four bulletproof windows. After checking her identification, a nurse behind the glass handed her a red plastic cup of liquid methadone, watched her drink it, and then asked her to state her name—a method of ensuring that patients swallowed the methadone, since it's hard to speak with liquid in your mouth.

MELISSA BEGAN HER methadone treatment like everyone else did, at "level one." That meant she was required to attend the methadone clinic daily, seven days per week. She frequently gave urine drug screens to prove consumption of methadone rather than diversion to the black market. After about two weeks of the physician slowly increasing the dose, her body adjusted to the methadone, and she felt her cravings for prescription pain pills diminish. Fortunately, so long as she took the methadone daily, she also didn't experience withdrawal symptoms. She did experience some sweating and constipation from the methadone, though these side effects were minimal compared to the ups and downs of chaotic drug use.

The methadone clinic also required Melissa to attend weekly group counseling and weekly individual counseling while she was at level one. Sometimes the group counseling sessions were helpful, especially if the group counselor listened rather than spoke down to the participants. But other times the groups were led by a young college student with no clear understanding of addiction and who read straight from a book. It was like story time for adults, and Melissa felt patronized.

Unfortunately, it took two months before Melissa could obtain an individual counseling session, which she felt would better address her mental health issues. For weeks she left notes under counselors' doors trying to get their attention, but the clinic had hundreds of patients and only a few counselors. And according to clinic rules, until Melissa could prove regular individual counseling attendance, she could not advance to level two, which would only require her to come to the clinic six days per week. She longed for one day per week when she could sleep in past three in the morning.

Finally, Melissa obtained an individual counseling appointment, but then she was quickly introduced to another problem—vanishing counselors. During her two years at the methadone clinic, Melissa saw seven individual counselors. By now I have heard so many stories of vanishing methadone clinic counselors that I'm surprised whenever a patient has the same counselor for more than a few months. Melissa described multiple instances of patients banging on the door while she was in the middle of a counseling session, desperate for their own sessions, prompting the counselor to check his or her watch. Eventually the clinic pasted signs on counselors' doors: "Do not knock while counseling is in session."

Melissa found the individual counseling sessions helpful but only when she liked the counselor. And given the high turnover rate, as soon as Melissa found a counselor whom she liked, that counselor disappeared. Furthermore, Melissa had no say in choosing the counselor to whom she was assigned. She even had two antimethadone counselors in the clinic who urged her to stop methadone treatment, telling her that methadone was not real recovery even though she no longer misused opioids. That's not as rare as you might think. In the course of writing this book, I have encountered other stories of anti-methadone counselors working in methadone clinics.

DURING HER TWO YEARS at the methadone clinic, Melissa obtained an online certificate in business management. She has no passion for business and in conversation still calls herself a nurse, even though she can no longer legally practice as one. With the business certificate, she obtained a position working for a retired anthropology professor who, despite retirement, was authoring a book. Describing the work, Melissa says, "Basically, I was his computer. He didn't know how to check or answer email." The position had low pay and no health benefits.

To be at the professor's house by eight o'clock every morning, Melissa had to provide the methadone clinic proof of her work, allowing her to dose early. Pay stubs were insufficient proof of employment; only a letter on employer letterhead addressed to the clinic would suffice. Fortunately, Melissa's employer was kind and understanding, but she fears that many people get fired just for requesting such a letter. I suspect that most employers don't realize substance use disorder is covered by the Americans with Disabilities Act.[167] In other words, it is illegal to fire an employee merely for having the disorder or participating in treatment unless that employee is still actively using drugs.[167] Not only are employers unlikely to know how the Americans with Disabilities Act applies to substance use disorder, employees are probably unaware as well. And employees in Melissa's position can rarely afford an attorney to advise them of their civil rights.

Eventually it was time for Melissa to move on to a new job. The professor had finished his book and was now truly retiring. With a letter of recommendation from the professor in hand, Melissa found a new job at her city's department of motor vehicles, a job with health benefits and promotion opportunities. But the office was very strict about timeliness, and Melissa felt extremely uncomfortable disclosing her addiction and methadone treatment to her supervisors. By now she had two take-home days of methadone, both on the weekend, but she was tired of driving to the methadone clinic each weekday before work. She racked her brain for other options.

Under federal and state law, she could obtain a prescription for methadone for *pain management* from any physician, nurse practitioner, or physician assistant. With such a prescription, she could legally acquire the medication from a regular local pharmacy on a monthly basis, rather than daily. Following the advice of a friend, Melissa wrote a heartfelt letter to a new nurse practitioner in a family medicine practice, just a few minutes' drive from Melissa's house. In the letter, Melissa described her car accident, her back pain, and her history of opioid addiction. She described her attendance at the methadone clinic, how she had to wake up daily at 3:00 a.m. to get in line to dose at 5:00 a.m., sometimes waiting in line for an hour, and then drive back to work. Melissa delivered the letter to the nurse practitioner's office. She didn't ask for anything in the letter, other than saying that she'd really appreciate an appointment. Expecting to hear nothing back, Melissa was surprised to receive a phone call stating that she had an appointment as a new patient.

A few days later, shaking like a leaf, Melissa visited the nurse practitioner. She repeated the story she'd told in her letter, again asking for nothing in particular. The woman looked Melissa squarely in the eyes and said, "I am going to write you a methadone prescription for your pain." But on the prescription pad, she wrote the dose and frequency of methadone given for addiction treatment, not pain. A few hours later, Melissa picked up a month's prescription at the local grocery store pharmacy.

To this day, Melissa does not know why the nurse practitioner did what she did. As far as Melissa could tell, she had no formal training or experience in addiction medicine. Maybe it was another example of nurse camaraderie. Melissa has no doubt that the woman prescribed methadone with addiction treatment in mind, although Melissa does believe that the methadone helps with her back pain as well. For almost a year, she continued receiving monthly methadone prescriptions "for pain" in this fashion.

Then one day, Melissa tried to make an appointment through the office's online patient portal but received no response. Worried, she walked into the family medicine practice and explained that she wanted an appointment with her nurse practitioner. The receptionist coolly stated that the nurse practitioner no longer worked there. In panic, Melissa asked if she could speak to the nurse practitioner's medical assistant. The receptionist said the medical assistant likewise no longer worked there. Shaking, Melissa explained that she was never told the nurse practitioner was leaving; she had not received a letter or any notice. The receptionist said not to worry, that they would reschedule Melissa with a new provider, a physician who had recently joined the practice.

A few days later, Melissa anxiously waited to meet her new provider in the examination room. When the physician arrived, before even saying hello or introducing himself, he exclaimed, "Just so you know, I don't prescribe methadone." Instead, he offered Melissa a referral to a pain management specialist and physical therapy. Back in her car, Melissa sobbed behind the steering wheel. She dreaded resuming her trips to the methadone clinic. Having quit the clinic over a year ago, she would have to start again at level one. In a panic, Melissa called her close friends, begging them for advice. She even briefly considered buying methadone off the street, but she feared it would trigger her to buy other substances, including Lortab.

For two weeks, Melissa struggled to prevent withdrawal symptoms and cravings using only the handful of methadone pills she had left. That meant skipping some doses or taking half doses. Then while at work one day she received a phone call from her friend Kendall with good news. Kendall, a licensed practical nurse, had carefully described Melissa's situation to her own supervisor, a psychiatrist, emphasizing Melissa's need for methadone treatment for both pain and addiction. The psychiatrist casually responded that he would accept

Melissa as a patient. Following the phone call, Melissa remembers going into the department of motor vehicles bathroom, getting into the fetal position, and crying tears of joy.

The psychiatrist later told Melissa that he would help her with her "pain," but that given the pressure from insurance companies and his administrators, he could only do so for a year, just enough to let her comfortably taper off the medication. That is Melissa's situation today. She is stable, she is comfortable, but she lives in fear, knowing that her next prescription might be her last. In the meantime, her city has approved the opening of a methadone clinic, but she has not heard any concrete plans. Every day she drives by the site on which it will supposedly be built, hoping to see construction workers. So far there are none. She worries that given the negativity in the local news media toward methadone clinics it might never open. But all she can do is remain hopeful.

METHADONE FOR ADDICTION treatment is arguably the most stringently regulated medication provided on an outpatient basis in the United States. It may only be administered and dispensed in opioid treatment programs (OTPs), also called methadone clinics. To dispense methadone, OTPs must be certified by the Substance Abuse and Mental Health Services Administration, accredited by a government-approved organization, registered with the Drug Enforcement Administration (DEA), and registered with the state in which they are located. While dispensing methadone, OTPs must follow a hodgepodge of federal and state regulations. For example, under federal law they can only dispense methadone to people with over one year of opioid addiction history unless the individual is pregnant, was recently incarcerated, or has previously been engaged in methadone treatment.[168] Some states go further, requiring patients to have more than two years of opioid addiction history before beginning methadone treatment.[169] These regulations do not apply to methadone used for pain management, despite the fact that methadone for addiction treatment is literally lifesaving—dramatically cutting the overdose death risk[23]—while the effectiveness of methadone for chronic pain management is largely inconclusive.[170] In fact, methadone for addiction treatment is one of the most rigorously evaluated and best studied medications in the entire field of medicine.[171]

Under federal law, patients must attend the OTP daily, with only one take-home dose permitted weekly during the first ninety days of methadone treatment.[168] At the end of one stable year, patients can obtain up to two weeks of take-home doses at a time.[168] The maximum take-home amount, a one-month supply, does not occur until after two years of stable methadone treatment.[168] These federal regulations create a floor on top of which states can add further restrictions. For example, Indiana permits a maximum of one week of take-home doses after one year of stabilization, unless the OTP petitions the government for an exemption for a particular patient.[172]

Even when patients have maximum take-home privileges, states can still subject them to random urine drug screens and bottle counts. Sherri, a young stay-at-home mother of three in North Carolina, has been stable for two years. She has full take-home privileges, meaning she can take home a month's worth of methadone. Yet her clinic still calls her in weekly for random bottle counts and urine drug screens, a tedious process since she must drive with her young children to a clinic one hour away on short notice.

When I first began interviewing people in methadone treatment, I fully expected to hear uniform complaints about daily clinic attendance requirements. But the reality is a bit more nuanced. Many, though not all, believe that the structure and accountability of daily attendance was critical at the beginning of their recovery. Some feel that daily attendance forced them to schedule their day around treatment rather than the ups and downs of heroin highs, though for employed people or parents of young children, the inflexible structure can prove more of a liability. Others emphasized the accountability benefits of methadone clinics permitting take-home doses only after stability has been reached. For example, when I asked Eric, a former injection drug user, whether he disagrees with daily dosing requirements, he said, "No, I think it's great. You got counseling and groups and it's kind of making me have to be responsible if you want to keep your medicine and take it home with you eventually, so you don't have to go every day." Similarly, Michael, who is in recovery in the Southeast, said, "I know that there's going to be consequences if I don't get up every day and go to the methadone clinic . . . it's a good thing for me right now. Not only that, but it keeps me accountable as well."

Relatedly, some patients express a sense of pride when they reach the next take-home level. Clinic physicians, nurses, and counselors can capitalize on this by praising people for their hard work. However, sometimes the different take-home levels prompt patients to express scorn toward patients at lower levels. For example, Sherri says, "The people who've been there as long as me, if not longer, that still go every day, seven days a week . . . I feel like that's kind of their fault; they're not doing what they need to do."

Daily dosing with take-homes permitted in a stepwise manner is based on a well-studied tool in addiction medicine: contingency management.[173] Simply put, contingency management means giving a reward in response to a specific behavior.[174] On its own, contingency management is usually insufficient for recovery. For example, it is ineffective to simply tell someone, "Each day that you don't use heroin, I'll give you twenty dollars." Why? Because the contingency management alone is not addressing the person's original reason for drug use, such as coping with childhood trauma, nor is it directly addressing physical cravings or withdrawal symptoms. But as a complement to treatment, contingency management can be an effective tool. For example, contingency management helps some people comply with treatment regimens, with the treatment then leading to stabilization. Essentially, daily methadone clinic attendance ensures consistent consumption of the medication, preventing physical highs and lows, enabling the individual to feel normal. When people feel physically stable, they can start to work on their underlying psychological problems.

But sometimes clinics create their own rules, not required by law, that prevent a patient who should be at a higher take-home level from ever reaching it. For example, some clinics prevent patients who use marijuana from ever advancing to the next level. Whether such a rule is appropriate is a contentious topic, both among patients and providers. For example, Jarrod had complete take-home privileges in Washington, but since moving to North Carolina a few years ago, he is still at level one because he continues to smoke marijuana. Likewise, Riley in the Midwest, believes he will never get take-home privileges at his clinic because of marijuana use: "It's just easier for me to smoke a little marijuana than to shove other pills down my throat, which I don't need. Why would I have to take antidepressants and antianxiety medication if I don't have to?" He finds the marijuana restriction ridiculous given his significant progress in methadone treatment. He says, "I'm a completely different person, people trust me right now. You know, people will leave me with their kids and stuff right now, but if I wasn't going to the methadone clinic, that would've never happened."

Regardless of whether patients can advance to higher levels of take-home privileges, clinics should not kick patients out for misusing opioids, missing appointments, or for using other drugs. At a minimum, clinics should keep these patients on daily doses at the clinic. Decades of studies clearly demonstrate that a stable methadone dose is a strong predictor of methadone treatment retention, and methadone treatment retention is a strong predictor of positive health outcomes.[120,175,176] When clinics fire patients, they virtually guarantee that former patients will resort to buying opioids on the street.[176] As compared to high-barrier methadone clinics, low-barrier methadone clinics, meaning ones that accept people still misusing opioids, using other drugs, or engaging in criminal activity, have demonstrated efficacy in decreasing HIV/AIDS risk behavior, heroin use, mortality, and criminal behavior.[176]

Would it be possible to eliminate daily clinic visits altogether, perhaps only requiring daily clinics for brand-new patients while dosing needs are determined? In fact, other countries, such as the United Kingdom and France, have methadone treatment models significantly less stringent than our own. A potential benefit of our current system of daily methadone dosing and laxer buprenorphine prescribing is that we allow people to self-sort into the most appropriate treatment regimen for their needs. For example, people with long-term injection drug use or serious co-occurring conditions may benefit from the enhanced structure and accountability of daily methadone clinic attendance, while those with shorter addiction histories or no serious co-occurring conditions may find less stringent buprenorphine treatment sufficient. Furthermore, methadone has stronger activity at the opioid receptors, so methadone may better manage cravings and prevent withdrawal symptoms in people with more severe opioid addiction, especially injection drug users and those with a long opioid addiction history.[12] And long-term drug users may have greater need of the ancillary services, structure, and accountability provided by methadone clinics.

Nevertheless, long-term daily clinic visits may be overkill for some clients. Sherri, like some interviewees, has mixed feelings about daily clinic visits, recognizing the accessibility problems they create. "You see people doing exactly everything you're supposed to do and going to all of the meetings and clean drug screens every time. And you know, it does feel good to earn those [take-homes]. But it does become a little bit of a problem, because you do have to wait such a long time to start getting take-homes. It does interfere with everyday life. I know some people have lost their jobs because the line was too long or they were on hold for some reason, and I do see that as a problem, and they tried to kind of fix that where you have early dosing if you prove you have a job. But dosing is usually at five o'clock and unfortunately a lot of people have to be at work at five thirty or six. I do know a lot of people that have lost jobs because either they couldn't [dose early] or they just were continually late." Additionally, clients who move from one state to another, or even from one clinic to another clinic in the same city, are often forced to restart at level one.

When federal or state regulations are too rigid, physicians lack the ability to create flexible treatment plans. One could envision a different regulatory model wherein the providers at the methadone clinic, a team of physicians and counselors, make regular, individualized assessments of patients' progress, on which they base take-home allowance, thereby potentially allowing monthlong take-home doses for some highly motivated, stable patients earlier than one year. Going a step further, one could envision a model wherein a stabilized patient can eventually switch to receiving methadone prescriptions outside of the methadone clinic, such as from a primary care physician and picking up the medication from a local pharmacy. This is similar to the model currently used in France successfully. In other words, one could envision a system that allows patients like Melissa to do exactly what Melissa does, except in an aboveboard, legal manner. After all, patients can already receive methadone for pain management from office-based providers. A US study exploring the potential transition of stabilized patients from methadone clinics to office-based primary care providers demonstrated high satisfaction among both patients and physicians.[177] In the study, the transition also improved physicians' perceptions of methadone treatment—supporting the argument that physicians' misconceptions about methadone are partly due to methadone treatment's separation from mainstream medicine.[177]

Such a flexible model would require significantly more clinic resources than are available today. Clinics would need to hire enough physicians and counselors to ensure regular, comprehensive patient progress evaluations on which flexible, evidence-based decision-making would be founded. But today so few addiction-trained physicians exist that such a model seems more theoretical than realistic. Significantly more physician training in addiction treatment in medical school and residency is needed, including more addiction medicine fellowships. Addiction medicine as a profession would need to be viewed more legitimately by fellow members of the medical profession[178] and the public than it is today. After all, addiction medicine only recently became a physician subspecialty, certified by the American Board of Preventive Medicine.[179]

Too often MAT providers are viewed as enablers who are harming rather than helping patients. When such stigma is coupled with low insurance reimbursement rates and the location of methadone clinics in disreputable parts of town, it is no wonder that few physicians seek work in methadone clinics. A flexible model would also require legislators and regulators to trust methadone providers more, granting individual clinics and providers greater autonomy over treatment decision-making—the kind of autonomy we already grant physicians in other areas of medicine.

Even though many methadone clinic patients appreciate the structure and accountability available within methadone clinics, they do not paint an altogether rosy picture of their experiences. Instead, people whom I have interviewed identify two serious, widespread problems with methadone clinics: limited clinic accessibility and lack of person-centered care. These same problems have been mentioned in regard to rural and urban clinics, in blue states and red states. I believe these problems are primarily a result of methadone clinics' stigma and separation from mainstream medicine, limiting health providers' and administrators' knowledge about and interest in opening new clinics. Few methadone clinics means limited competition between clinics, resulting in patients being stuck with whatever care they receive, even if it is provided without compassion and respect for patient preferences. Understandably, a patient already driving two hours daily to the nearest clinic won't switch to a clinic four hours away, even if that clinic provides more person-centered care.

Between 2003 and 2015, the number of methadone clinics barely grew, despite an increase in the number of patients receiving methadone treatment at preexisting clinics.[180] Most states have fewer than ten methadone clinics, with one state, Wyoming, lacking a single clinic.[91] Methadone clinics are also more likely to exist in urban rather than rural areas. With such limited availability, daily clinic visits become infeasible for patients who must travel long distances, waking up at ungodly hours if they have any hope of maintaining employment.

Like Melissa, they describe daily two-hour drives to and from the methadone clinic, especially in rural areas where public transportation is largely unavailable. Many people drive long distances to methadone clinics without drivers' licenses, which they have lost due to drug-related criminal charges. Methadone clinic patients so frequently lack drivers' licenses that several interviewees have described police waiting outside their clinics, eager to pull drivers over to ask for their IDs. Not willing to risk getting caught driving without a license, others rely on family members or friends to transport them daily. Mary Beth, who lives in Indiana, describes waking up daily at 4:00 a.m. to drive her twenty-one-year-old son an hour each way to the methadone clinic before beginning her work for an insurance company. She repeats this routine rain or shine, weekday or weekend, because her son's probation terms prohibit motor vehicle operation, and no reliable public transportation exists in their area. She does not remember the last day she slept in.

Person-centered care is also rarely experienced in methadone clinics. Perhaps except for within the Veterans Health Administration, methadone clinic patients do not describe feeling like they are attending a medical facility, especially when forced to wait in long, winding lines with receptionists and nurses behind bulletproof glass counting piles of cash. Vanishing counselors and limited counselor choice further deprive patients of the feeling that they are just that—patients—rather than "junkies" undeserving of quality care.

Eric explained how suddenly losing a counselor with whom you have established a therapeutic relationship can be extremely difficult: "I know people where they lost a counselor and it triggered them. They used again. I wish the [methadone clinics] paid their counselors better or made it a better work environment where the counselors will want to stay." Describing the limited counseling accessibility in her methadone clinic, Christina, who lives in the Southeast, said, "If you want to get clean, you can, but you have to try really hard because it almost feels like it's kind of rigged against you. Like everything you [get] is not quite the right help that you need, and you just kind of have to focus on yourself and say you want this enough."

The combination of counselors' inadequate MAT education and their own recovery through twelve-step programs can also create a fertile breeding ground for misconceptions about MAT efficacy. Not surprisingly, few addiction counselors are eager to work in methadone clinics. Nevertheless, methadone clinic patients often describe individual counseling as very beneficial to their recovery, especially if they have a history of trauma.

Despite its efficacy, and almost fifty years after its introduction in the United States, methadone treatment is still publicly stigmatized. Clinic locations hardly help. Brooke, who is in recovery, says, "They're always just kind of nasty places to go to on the bad side of town. It's in an undesirable location and it makes you feel like an undesirable to be there." Often located in crime-ridden areas, methadone clinics are an easy target for blame if any crime occurs. Yet, methadone treatment has been repeatedly associated with decreasing criminal activity.[23,181]

I routinely ask people in recovery how they would characterize methadone clinic patients, and I have received a fascinating divide in responses. Current or former methadone clinic patients usually believe that most people go to methadone clinics for the "right" reasons—to stop opioid misuse or at least to stop feeling sick, meaning to stop withdrawal symptoms. The latter should not be dismissed as an illegitimate reason for methadone treatment: *not* feeling sick can jump-start a desire for complete recovery, something difficult to think about amid strong cravings and withdrawal symptoms.

In contrast, people in recovery who have never participated in methadone treatment frequently view it negatively. Describing antimethadone stigma in her community, Sherri says, "In every single [counseling] group I've ever been to [at the methadone clinic], at least one person brings it up, saying, 'My boyfriend doesn't understand why I'm here and I don't know why I can't dose out faster.' It's very misunderstood by everybody, and you can see how much people are affected by [stigma], especially when a significant other doesn't understand about it. My boyfriend, when I first got with him a year ago, I was straight up honest with him, I said, 'I'm a recovering heroin addict. I go to the methadone clinic.' I took him with me and he went to a couple of my counseling sessions. . . . That really helped him understand what was going on and [now] he's super supportive of me."

Even some buprenorphine treatment patients look down on methadone clinic patients. One methadone clinic patient points to the following reasons for the discrepancy: the word "buprenorphine" sounds more medical than "methadone," which incidentally sounds like "meth," as in crystal meth, and buprenorphine is provided by regular office-based physicians, often in nice parts of town, rather than methadone clinics in seedy areas. Furthermore, some interviewees point to the inability to feel heroin if taken during buprenorphine treatment, while claiming that you might still feel heroin if used during methadone treatment when the methadone dose is too low.

Interviewees with methadone treatment experience argue that an appropriate methadone dose is critical to treatment success. Yet over 40 percent of US methadone clinic patients receive too *low* a dosage, with nonwhite minorities particularly likely to receive insufficient doses.[182] Significant evidence exists that methadone treatment programs should provide a minimum dose of 80 mg/day, as methadone dose is strongly related to treatment effectiveness.[183–185] Not only do higher methadone doses better prevent cravings, but the higher the methadone dose, the less likely the individual is to feel the effects of other opioids, such as heroin.[186] For example, a small double-blind study found that people cannot distinguish heroin from a placebo if they have an appropriate dose of methadone in their system.[186] Christina told me, "There was one time in the first year [of methadone treatment] when after the first week, I slipped up and went and bought some heroin and I didn't feel a damn thing. I was so mad. I was like, wow, I let myself relapse for nothing." I asked if someone could feel heroin despite undergoing methadone treatment, and she said, "If you're dosing pretty low, I think maybe, yeah, you can still feel it, but not nearly as strong as you could when you aren't taking methadone."

Low methadone doses are not evidence-based; instead, they are likely a reflection of some clinic owners' or providers' anti–harm reduction attitudes.[182] Like Christina, Blaine explained that during the first few days of methadone treatment he continued to use heroin, because the clinic started him on the low dose of 20 mg/day, despite many years of heroin use and his high tolerance for opioids. Not surprisingly, he still had cravings. It wasn't until the clinic increased his dose sufficiently that he stopped using heroin. I asked how he feels about methadone clinics starting people on very low doses. He responded, "With 'go low and go slow' it's taken way too many people too long to get comfortable. So, of course, if I'm not comfortable, what am I going to do? I'm going to do what I always know makes me feel better and I'm going to get high."

After months of methadone treatment, Blaine feels normal, with no cravings for heroin and no euphoria from methadone. Interestingly, he claims that those who feel euphoria from methadone either have a very low tolerance, and possibly shouldn't be undergoing methadone treatment to begin with, or else they are taking very high doses of methadone purchased off of the street. The vast majority of methadone sold on the street, and methadone-related overdose deaths,[187] consist of pain management prescriptions diverted to the black market. Methadone prescriptions for pain management are in pill form rather than liquid form and are provided at a different dosage and frequency than in methadone clinics. Bryan, another interviewee, admitted that when he first started methadone treatment for addiction, prior to fully committing to recovery, he considered selling some of his daily doses. But after racking his brains, he could not formulate a way to get the daily doses out of the clinic, saying, "Believe me, if there was a way to game the system, I would have figured it out."

Methadone diversion is also very misunderstood. Studies suggest a wide range of reasons why people illicitly buy and sell methadone. For example, some people sell part of their own methadone to supplement their low incomes or to afford the cash necessary to pay cash-only methadone clinics. Some provide friends or relatives with methadone to prevent withdrawal symptoms as an altruistic gesture, especially if friends or relatives cannot access a clinic.[181,188–190] Patients may buy street methadone to supplement too low doses from their clinic or simply because they cannot access the clinic due to financial or transportation reasons.[181,188–190] In other words, the reasons for methadone street sales can be far more complex than the stereotype of nefarious drug dealers helping users get high. In light of methadone treatment's clear, well-studied benefits, legal restrictions to prevent diversion or misuse should be balanced in favor of helping people access lifesaving treatment.

The lack of person-centered care, high patient-provider ratios, and publicly visible lines of often shabbily dressed people persuade the public that methadone is a bad treatment—even though it's really the provision of methadone rather than the medication itself that is so problematic. It is, therefore, unsurprising that politicians can be vehemently anti–methadone treatment. But even the most anti-methadone politician might change his or her mind if made aware of methadone treatment's fiscal benefits. Both methadone and buprenorphine are cost-effective,[23,191,192] saving taxpayer money on health care services, social services, and law enforcement. Interestingly, researchers believe that methadone expansion is even more cost-effective than buprenorphine expansion, but methadone treatment is less likely to expand quickly given the strict regulatory environment in which methadone clinics operate, one in which opening a new clinic or even keeping an existing clinic open can feel like a minefield.[191] For example, one medical director of a Florida methadone clinic described having to appear before local lawmakers annually to argue the case for keeping his clinic open. The arguments always feel like an uphill battle, despite the number of patients the clinic is helping.

EVEN THOUGH METHADONE, and increasingly buprenorphine, is the medical standard of care for treating pregnant women with opioid addiction,[23] many medical professionals and the public lack this knowledge. Sherri, the stay-at-home mother of three, recently formed a Facebook-based support group for mothers undergoing methadone treatment. Her personal experience prompted her to do so.

She had been undergoing methadone treatment for about three years when she became pregnant with her first child, Rose. Encouraged by her ob-gyn to stop methadone treatment because it might increase the baby's risk of being born with neonatal abstinence syndrome, Sherri quit cold turkey. Her ob-gyn was proud. But while experiencing methadone withdrawal symptoms, Sherri miscarried and lost her baby. She was so depressed that she returned to heroin use. For a time, it made her feel emotionally numb, exactly what she wanted, but soon her life started spiraling out of control. When her husband threatened to leave her, she restarted treatment at the methadone clinic. Sherri considers the four-month gap between quitting and restarting methadone the worst time of her life. Not only did she lose her baby, she feels she lost years of progress in recovery. In tears, she explained that her ob-gyn wasn't the only one who pressured her to quit methadone treatment; her mother and sister did too, saying that only a terrible mother would continue methadone treatment while pregnant. Sherri's experience reflects widespread misconceptions about methadone treatment during pregnancy.

Babies born to mothers undergoing methadone treatment will not necessarily have neonatal abstinence syndrome, a condition in which the baby experiences painful withdrawals from the opioid, much the same way an adult does upon quitting opioids.[181] Furthermore, babies born to mothers undergoing methadone treatment have comparable developmental outcomes to babies in control groups.[23] The treatment for neonatal abstinence syndrome is actually very low doses of methadone or morphine provided in the neonatal intensive care unit.[193] Videos of babies with neonatal abstinence syndrome are heartbreaking; the babies' muscles have uncontrollable spasms as they scream in pain. But while the public fears mothers taking methadone, what they really should fear is mothers quitting methadone as medically prescribed and relapsing to oxycodone, heroin, or fentanyl misuse, virtually guaranteeing not only neonatal abstinence syndrome but a particularly severe form of the condition.[120]

Importantly, methadone helps stabilize the lifestyle of the woman, and therefore the home of the forthcoming child. Untreated or ineffectively treated opioid misuse in pregnant women increases the risk of unstable housing, financial hardship, physical abuse, lack of prenatal care, and communicable disease acquisition, all of which can harm the child.[194] In contrast, methadone treatment of the pregnant woman significantly improves maternal, fetal, and neonatal outcomes in comparison with nonpharmacological treatment only.[195]

When Sherri became pregnant with her next child, Autumn, she decided to continue methadone treatment, closely monitored by a different ob-gyn in collaboration with her methadone clinic physician. When Autumn was born, she had no neonatal abstinence symptoms and went home after a few days in the hospital. Sherri's ob-gyn also encouraged her to breastfeed, something that is safe to do while a mother is undergoing methadone treatment.[194]

MANY PEOPLE WHO BEGIN methadone treatment have no desire to stop, especially if it has helped them stabilize an otherwise chaotic life. They stay at a stable dose for years. Others desire only short-term methadone treatment and slowly taper off the medication after achieving stability. Among people who taper off methadone, some eventually decide to switch to buprenorphine treatment, thereby necessitating a manhunt for the nearest buprenorphine treatment provider who is sometimes only slightly easier to find than a methadone clinic.

Patients who switch to buprenorphine must undergo partial detoxification, a difficult process in which they will experience withdrawal symptoms for a few days, though not nearly as many days of withdrawal symptoms as switching to extended-release naltrexone. When I ask methadone clinic patients whether they have considered switching to buprenorphine given the less stringent regulations on buprenorphine, the most common response I get is fear of withdrawal symptoms associated with the detoxification process. Eric says, "You've got to come off [methadone] completely. It'd be like two, three days I think before we can start Suboxone. I'm not in the right mind-set yet, it scares the crap out of me." Without palliative care for painful withdrawal symptoms, patients are at risk of relapse.

Palliative care could theoretically be inpatient, though this rarely occurs given that insurance almost never covers inpatient medical management of opioid withdrawal symptoms. Palliative care could also be outpatient, something insurance is more likely to cover. Methadone clinics have the infrastructure to provide this outpatient care. But while methadone clinics are adept at tapering people down to the minimum methadone dose, they often neglect to help people make the complete transition to buprenorphine or extended-release naltrexone, especially when clinics don't offer buprenorphine or extended-release naltrexone treatment. In a recent report, the Substance Abuse and Mental Health Services Administration stated that few opioid treatment programs supervise a complete methadone withdrawal process, partially due to fears that individuals will relapse, with relapse leading to overdose.[196] But without such supervision, methadone clinic patients have difficulty switching to other forms of MAT if they choose to do so. Even though the Substance Abuse and Mental Health Services Administration urges OTPs to offer all forms of MAT,[196] in 2015 only slightly more than half offered buprenorphine and less than a quarter offered extended-release naltrexone, demonstrating not only the level of separation between mainstream medicine and OTPs but also between the treatment tools available.[180] As a result, people wishing to switch medications are usually in the unenviable position of managing their own withdrawal symptoms. Realizing that she might relapse during the withdrawal process, one woman described asking her family to lock her in the basement, thereby preventing her from seeking heroin on the street that could immediately ease withdrawal symptoms during her transition to buprenorphine.

SYSTEMATIC REVIEWS of decades of rigorous randomized controlled trials,[92,101] including multisite longitudinal studies from multiple continents,[197] leave no doubt that methadone is more effective than nonpharmacological treatments alone, such as counseling, at decreasing opioid misuse, opioid overdose rates, criminal activity, and HIV/AIDS risk behaviors, such as drug injection.[23] Methadone is the most comprehensively and rigorously studied form of addiction treatment with the largest evidence base.[23] Like buprenorphine, methadone for addiction treatment is listed by the World Health Organization as an "essential medicine," meaning it should be widely available across all nations given its significant health benefits.[198] Nevertheless, people in recovery and their families, politicians, health care providers, and the public are often either adamantly against methadone or on the fence about its effectiveness. Widespread myths about the medication coupled with poor services make the stigma difficult to overcome.

Myths associated with the medication circulate within recovery communities, including among people participating in other forms of MAT. One of the most common myths is that methadone "gets in your bones." Another one is that it "rots your teeth." But as multiple physicians have explained to me, people in active drug use often don't take good care of their teeth, sometimes for decades. In fact, one addictionologist said the first physical trait he notices during new patient appointments is teeth, as teeth can indicate drug use severity. Once patients are stabilized on methadone, they sometimes visit a dentist for the first time in years, maybe in their entire lives, where they discover tooth decay, which they then mistakenly attribute to methadone rather than long-term poor hygiene.

Another myth is that the medication turns people into "zombies," causing them to nod off throughout the day, rendering them unable to focus on tasks or operate motor vehicles. While it is true that inappropriately high doses of methadone could make someone nod off, an individual undergoing methadone treatment at an appropriate dose with adequate monitoring will act and feel normal. Of course, if an opioid-naïve person or an intermittent opioid user with relatively low tolerance starts methadone treatment, then they will likely feel euphoria or nod off given their lack of tolerance. But under federal law, methadone clinics can only treat people with one or more years of opioid use disorder—a point at which low tolerance is very unlikely. For people with less than a year of opioid use disorder, buprenorphine or extended-release naltrexone are great treatment options—that is, if they can find a physician prescribing those medications.

5

THE ELUSIVE ADDICTION-TREATING PHYSICIAN

KELLIE HAD EXPERIMENTED with a variety of drugs as an adolescent but had never been hooked on anything. Ten years later, as a mother of three young kids and in a violent relationship with her boyfriend, she injected heroin to help her relax. Soon it was all she could think about. She loved her children, but heroin clouded everything. Each morning she would wake up wanting to quit, *intending* to quit, but within a few hours she was shooting up again. One day, Kellie's sister, Monique, found the children hungry, dirty, and crying in a house littered with needles. Monique took the kids to her own house, telling Kellie she would give her a chance to "get straight" before notifying the state's Department of Child Services.

Wanting help, Kellie voluntarily checked herself into a local detoxification center. During the few days of detox, she felt such overwhelming cravings that she could think of only one thing—her next hit of heroin. The moment she left detox, she drove straight to her dealer. In response, Monique contacted the Department of Child Services, who formally removed Kellie's children and placed them in Monique's care.

Once more, Kellie voluntarily entered detox. Once more, after detox the facility gave her a few brochures but made no effort to connect her to ongoing treatment. Therefore, Kellie took matters into her own hands and drove to the large community mental health and addiction treatment center downtown. She asked for addiction treatment, explaining that she had just completed detox but still felt cravings and was deeply depressed. Even though the facility technically allowed walk-ins, the approximately two-hour wait merely resulted in a rudimentary evaluation, after which Kellie was told she would receive a phone call to schedule an appointment. About a week later, Kellie did receive a phone call, but the receptionist explained that group counseling was full and was required prior to sessions with an individual counselor. The handful of staff psychiatrists was also not accepting new patients. Kellie hung up in tears.

A few hours later, she injected heroin on the bathroom floor. She thought about killing herself by purposely overdosing. The next few weeks were a blur. She did not want to get high; she just wanted to survive the next few hours. Seeing her misery, a friend undergoing Suboxone treatment with a local primary care physician offered one of his own strips. He said it would at least prevent the sickness of heroin withdrawals. A few days later, Kellie took the Suboxone and felt better almost immediately. She did not feel high, merely normal, a feeling she had not had in a long time. The friend warned her not to use heroin in the immediate future or else the Suboxone in her system would interact negatively with the heroin, making her sick.

The next day, Kellie bought another strip from the same friend, though the friend raised the price significantly. Remembering how the Suboxone made her feel, Kellie decided to start treatment on her own. She tried calling her friend's Suboxone-prescribing physician to schedule an appointment. But the receptionist immediately said the physician was not accepting new patients. Kellie asked for a recommendation to another Suboxone provider in the area. The receptionist did not know of any, but she encouraged Kellie to find a list of buprenorphine prescribers on the Substance Abuse and Mental Health Services Administration's website.

Kellie entered her zip code into the government website and found four other buprenorphine-prescribing physicians in her city.

Her heart raced with the anticipation of help that was in sight. She called the first physician: not accepting new patients. She called the second physician: no longer prescribing buprenorphine. She called the third physician: his office didn't even seem to know what buprenorphine was. Finally, with a sinking feeling, she learned that the fourth physician had retired.

Still determined to get help, Kellie expanded her online search to physicians located within a one hundred–mile radius. Fortunately, the first listing in a neighboring city resulted in an appointment for the following week. The only downside? It was over an hour away. But Kellie didn't care. She could wait one week, so long as her friend kept selling her some of his own strips in the meantime.

ABOUT A QUARTER OF URBAN US counties and more than half of rural counties lack a single DATA-waivered physician,[199] meaning a physician who is legally able to prescribe buprenorphine under the Drug Addiction Treatment Act of 2000.*

In 2019, buprenorphine prescribers are still heavily restricted. A DATA-waivered physician can prescribe buprenorphine for up to thirty patients at one time during the first year of the DATA waiver, and then for up to one hundred patients thereafter. A small minority of physicians who operate in "qualified settings" or are board certified in addiction medicine can prescribe it for up to 275 patients beginning in their third year.[83] It is clear that these restrictions are based not so much on the medication's efficacy and safety potential, but rather on misunderstandings of the population that seeks buprenorphine treatment for addiction. Why else would the restrictions not apply to prescribing oxycodone or hydrocodone?

---

* Note that having a DATA-waivered physician in your county does not mean that buprenorphine is actually accessible, merely that at least one physician is legally able to prescribe it. Whether he or she prescribes it, is accepting new patients, and accepts your insurance are totally different matters.

Many experts in the early 2000s viewed the medication's FDA approval as a turning point in addiction health services. Office-based prescribing could dramatically expand treatment accessibility. It might even lead to patients feeling more comfortable discussing opioid addiction with their primary care physicians, who for the first time since the passage of the Harrison Act could prescribe something useful for opioid addiction treatment from their offices rather than just referring patients to an outside provider.

But by 2015, fewer than half of US counties had a single DATA-waivered physician.[93] In 2018, more than a third of all US counties lacked a single DATA-waivered practitioner, and more than half of all rural counties lacked one.[200] Furthermore, many practitioners with a DATA waiver rarely prescribe buprenorphine to any patients.[201,202] One study found that a third of providers with a thirty-patient limit never prescribe the medication;[203] another found that almost half of DATA-waivered practitioners prescribe to fewer than five patients.[201]

Hoping to help patients locate a buprenorphine prescriber, the Substance Abuse and Mental Health Services Administration created an online public registry of DATA-waivered physicians. But even when physicians are listed on the government registry, they may have already met their maximum number of legal patients. And furthermore, physicians can opt out of the registry, resulting in a public list with only about half of DATA-waivered physicians visible.[202] Physicians tell me they opt out of the public list because they do not want to be known as the "Suboxone doctor." They do not want "unsavory" patients lining up outside their door, causing their more "respectable" patients to leave the practice. Some physicians prefer to prescribe buprenorphine to only a few trusted, handpicked patients. I have trouble imagining physicians in other health care fields hiding their practice in this way.

Like methadone, buprenorphine can technically be prescribed for pain at a different dosage and frequency, with patient limits and education requirements not applying to pain prescriptions, resulting in two parallel regulatory structures: one for stigmatized addiction patients and one more sympathetic to pain management patients. Many patients whom I have interviewed view buprenorphine patient limits as hypocritical and unfair. Ian said, "It's infuriating . . . they have [patient limits for buprenorphine], but not Opana or Oxycontin? That doesn't make any sense . . . why are you going to regulate the treatment and then not regulate the Oxycontin? . . . I know it gets in the way of people getting better because I [work at a syringe exchange] and probably once a week I get a call from someone saying, 'I'm looking for a Suboxone doctor,' and it's a whole ordeal because you have to find someone who has a space open and who takes Medicaid or a sliding scale."

Taking into account current medication-assisted treatment laws and prescriber capacity, approximately three times as many patients could receive buprenorphine treatment as are currently receiving methadone treatment, making buprenorphine treatment expansion a focus of some scholars and policy makers.[202] Nevertheless, buprenorphine treatment capacity, meaning the number of DATA-waivered physicians who can treat patients with buprenorphine, is far too low. In 2015, almost every state (96 percent), including the District of Columbia, had an opioid misuse rate higher than its buprenorphine treatment capacity.[202] Why is capacity so low? Stated differently, why do so few physicians have a DATA waiver? And of those who do, why do so few prescribe buprenorphine?

It is worth noting that buprenorphine is not the only difficult-to-access form of office-based MAT. Relatively few people in recovery from opioid addiction have tried extended-release naltrexone even though it does not activate the brain's opioid receptors, has relatively lower stigma than methadone and buprenorphine, and is subject to minimal regulations, with no patient limits or required special education for physicians. Ironically, the inability to divert the medication and sell it on the street has likely limited knowledge of extended-release naltrexone, since many in recovery report learning of buprenorphine by seeing it bought and sold illictly.[178] But among those patients who want to try extended-release naltrexone, the experience of finding a provider for that medication can be just as grueling and disheartening as finding a buprenorphine treatment provider.

OPIOID ADDICTION IS A relapsing health condition not dissimilar in treatment success rates from hypertension, asthma, and diabetes.[204] Yet people are far more likely to visit their physicians if they have hypertension, asthma, or diabetes than if they have an addiction. Instead, they think of physicians as an addiction treatment provider of last resort or are unsure what help a physician could provide at all. Self-help groups, such as Alcoholics Anonymous or Narcotics Anonymous, are by far the most common "treatment" setting, even though support groups do not say they provide treatment.[98] Never have I heard an interviewee say, "*When I realized I needed help with my addiction, I contacted my primary care physician*."

Consider how unusual it would be for a patient with any other deadly, chronic medical condition to first visit peer-led, nonprofessional support groups, then rehab centers (often with few, if any, physicians), and then counselors—all before finally contacting a physician. Furthermore, imagine that once the patient finally decided to contact a physician, the patient discovered that his primary care physician, like other physicians in the area, does not treat the condition with the latest evidence-based treatments. Instead, the physician merely refers the patient back to support groups, rehab centers, and counselors.

During the course of my research, I have conducted in-depth, semistructured interviews with dozens of physicians who provide addiction treatment. In one of my studies, I explicitly asked physicians to compare barriers to prescribing the oral versions of buprenorphine, such as Suboxone, and extended-release naltrexone (i.e., Vivitrol).[178] But I quickly realized I was asking the wrong question.

Barriers do not just exist to prescribing MAT; barriers exist to treating addiction, period. As a result, many physicians don't treat addiction at all, regardless of medication options. So, I changed my research question to: Why do so few office-based physicians, meaning those outside of methadone clinics or hospitals, treat addiction using any method?

It quickly became clear that physicians lack sufficient training in and education about addiction medicine. As a result, they fail to see themselves as addiction treatment providers. Instead, they feel that addiction treatment is the exclusive realm of counselors, support groups, and rehabilitation centers. According to one recent study of medical students' attitudes concerning addiction patients, the researchers found that "[the medical students] rarely mentioned addiction treatment, and when they did, they perceived it as something that was done by specialized counselors out in the community. At most, they perceived that the physicians' role was to identify and refer."[205] The problem is not that physicians collaborate with other professionals on addiction treatment teams. In fact, the larger and more interdisciplinary the team, the better! The problem is that physicians purposely exclude themselves from the interdisciplinary team or, at most, take a minor role.[206] But only physicians, nurse practitioners, and physician assistants can prescribe buprenorphine or extended-release naltrexone. And many states require that DATA-waivered nurse practitioners and physician assistants prescribing buprenorphine be supervised by a DATA-waivered physician.[207]

Medical schools and residency programs notoriously provide inadequate training in addiction medicine. In the words of Dr. Richardson, an internal medicine resident who only recently graduated from a major public university's medical school, "It's very minimal. I don't remember any formal lecture about addiction medicine at all." These feelings are pervasive and reported by multiple studies of medical school students.[208] One recent survey of internal medicine residents found that 37 percent reported having received *no* medical school addiction instruction; of the 63 percent who had some addiction training, only 47 percent received more than a single lecture, and only 25 percent interacted with an addiction patient.[209] Failure to provide more robust addiction training is inexcusable, particularly in the face of the opioid overdose epidemic. Some could argue that it amounts to educational malpractice.

Even when medical school curricula incorporate addiction medicine, it is rarely taught as an entire course,[210] instead comprising a much smaller niche, often a single lecture—grossly inadequate in light of the number of patients with addiction whom physicians will eventually see. Such meager education offerings send a loud message to medical students that addiction medicine is beneath them, unimportant, or irrelevant, despite the fact that 10 percent of their patients will experience a substance use disorder at some point in their lives.[211] In one interview, Dr. Johnson complained about the many hours her medical studies devoted to rare genetic diseases versus the single lecture on addiction, despite the fact that patients with rare genetic diseases are exactly that—rare. But rare genetic disorders hold educators' interest more than addiction science, which seems more pedestrian. She felt utterly unprepared for the many patients she would eventually see with opioid addiction.

Another internal medical resident, Dr. Palmer, had only been exposed to addiction medicine during a family medicine rotation through informal conversations with a family medicine physician who happened to have a board certification in addiction medicine. Addiction medicine was not even taught during Dr. Palmer's psychiatry rotation: "I guess [the psychiatry rotation] is tailored toward everything except addiction medicine because that's not on the shelf exam at the end of each rotation . . . and the stuff you learn is just sort of in passing, if you are having a conversation with one of your attendings."

Nor are these educational deficits remedied during residency. One recent study found that 25 percent of internal medical residents felt unprepared to diagnose addiction, and 62 percent felt unprepared to treat addiction; no resident reported feeling "very prepared."[209] In another study of over one hundred medical residents, none answered all questions about addiction medicine science and treatments correctly, almost half couldn't identify how buprenorphine treatment works on the brain, and 81 percent failed a naltrexone question; only 6 percent of residents correctly answered all MAT questions.[212] In light of these educational deficits, it is unsurprising that physicians report feeling less comfortable prescribing medications for addiction than prescribing medications for other chronic conditions.[213]

Dr. O'Brien, director of a large medical school's psychiatry residency program, disclosed that until a few years ago, the school's training in addiction medicine was limited to observations of twelve-step groups and a brief lecture. He strongly disagreed with this educational plan and advocated incorporating education about MAT, modern counseling methods, and other evidence-based treatment approaches. The prior minimal education implied that addiction treatment is not a matter for physicians but something left to support groups or counselors only.

Moreover, medical residents' exposure to addiction treatment typically occurs in short-term hospital or acute care settings rather than in other more representative settings, such as outpatient clinics. The fact that residents usually see addiction treatment in brief episodes is particularly unfortunate: they cannot witness how addiction treatment works over time, even though addiction is a chronic, relapsing disease. Without this long-term view, residents may assume that addiction treatment does not work. Nor do residents in short-term treatment settings learn how to adjust addiction treatments in response to patient progress or setbacks, or how to transition patients to different medications.

Inadequate addiction medicine education in medical schools and residency programs reflects the fact that very few medical school faculty members are trained in addiction medicine. Yet, both curriculum instruction and education through attending physicians contribute to a physician's perception of how effectively she can treat addiction. Moreover, addiction medicine faculty can serve as role models for students and residents, teaching them how—and how not—to interact with patients with addiction symptoms, lessons that few are currently learning.

We know that addiction medicine education works—specifically, that it increases physicians' preparedness to diagnose and manage addiction.[208] The best curricula will incorporate several features, including student exposure to patients in long-term treatment and recovery programs, student engagement in clinical work under the supervision of physicians experienced in treating addiction, and information on evidence-based treatment methods. Given the strong association between addiction, chronic pain,[214] and mental health disorders, addiction medicine education should explore the treatment intersection between these topics. In fact, about half of people who experience a substance use disorder will experience a mental health disorder during their lifetime, and vice versa.[215] Online training can also fill curriculum gaps, including programs that walk students through case vignettes in the style of "choose your own adventure." Such training methods can dramatically increase students' perceptions of addiction treatment effectiveness.[216]

Interestingly, the eight-hour course required for physicians to receive a DATA waiver, and thus to prescribe buprenorphine, can heighten their confidence in treating addiction and their willingness to do so.[212] Therefore, one potential route to expanding buprenorphine prescribing is to require this course, which is available online, in most residency programs regardless of whether a physician has a preexisting desire to treat addiction. For example, Dr. Capone's psychiatry fellowship required fellows to obtain DATA waivers for prescribing buprenorphine. Although an unusual requirement, she believes it should be universal. She stated, "At the end of the day, it's going to be a [general practitioner], it's going be a family practice, it's going to be the emergency room that sees the majority of these patients. So, I would like those three, in addition to psychiatry, to have [the buprenorphine certification course] as part of their training being mandatory. And in my ideal world they would all get buprenorphine waivers, so the burden doesn't fall on one person." This last statement reflects the fact that Dr. Capone is the only physician prescribing buprenorphine in her large treatment facility, which has hundreds of patients with opioid addiction. Eight hours, though, is arguably not enough time to address an immensely complex topic. It barely scratches the surface, but at least it is a start.

Given the United States' current and future public health needs, the woeful state of addiction education in medical schools and residency programs is indefensible. But there are few direct incentives to remedy these shortcomings. Medical schools must remain solvent, and relative to other fields of medicine, addiction medicine is not a profitable field. Addiction medicine is low-tech and thus less "sexy" than surgery or other fields that receive constant influxes of private donations and grant money. For medical schools to expand curricula and hire faculty experts, federal and state governments must increase targeted funding for addiction medicine education, and private donors must be persuaded of addiction medicine education's value—a tall order given that medical schools themselves often discount its importance.

But there is another way to motivate professional interest in addiction medicine: by increasing the number of addiction medicine questions on state medical licensing exams. To a large extent these tests dictate what is taught and what is studied. While "teaching to the test" is rarely the best educational strategy, tests should reflect the subjects on which professionals must be competent to practice, and addiction medicine surely meets that standard. Recent medical school graduates tell me that addiction medicine would receive greater educational attention if state medical licensing boards included the subject matter on exams. Medical schools care deeply about what percentage of students pass state licensing exams because the passage rates affect school rankings. But for addiction medicine to receive higher priority on these tests, members of state licensing boards must accord it higher significance, presenting the same dilemma that makes medical school educational reform so difficult.

Reforming medical school and residency programs, though, is not enough to remedy physicians' lack of knowledge. After all, most practicing physicians have passed those educational milestones. For physicians already working in office-based practices, mentoring is one well-regarded method for transferring knowledge and skills. The government created a Physician Clinical Support System for buprenorphine treatment, which is an educational support system geared toward non–addiction specialists who have already undergone the mandatory eight-hour training. It's a national network of trained physician-support mentors and includes phone, email, and in-person support.[217] The problem is that few of the physicians whom I have interviewed, even those already DATA-waivered, have heard of it. Mandatory continuing medical education on the topic, at least for physicians practicing in certain fields, could help. Another option is "academic detailing," basically a practice wherein health care practitioners trained by academics visit office-based physicians and promote certain underused treatments, much as a pharmaceutical representative would do, though with far less bias and no financial conflict of interest. While understudied in the context of addiction health services, existing research shows that academic detailing has promising results in increasing health care practitioner utilization of evidence-based treatment methods.[218] Similarly, the existence of state clinical guidelines for providing buprenorphine treatment is associated with more DATA-waivered physicians,[219] possibly because such guidelines increase physician education and confidence in addiction treatment.

Arguably all practicing physicians should be targeted with education efforts, but two groups stand out: primary care physicians and psychiatrists. The former is the most accessible group of physicians in the United States, and the latter is particularly well suited to address complex co-occurring mental health issues. Disconcertingly, some physicians whom I have interviewed seem to think that only psychiatrists should treat addiction. Yet, research indicates that people without severe co-occurring psychiatric conditions, such as post-traumatic stress disorder, or polysubstance use, such as both opioid use disorder and cocaine use disorder, do well in addiction treatment with a primary care physician or internist.[220] Though such patients may greatly benefit from meeting with a psychiatrist, all patients do not necessarily need addiction treatment from one—an important point given the paucity of psychiatrists in the United States and the existing stigma related to seeing a psychiatrist. An individual obtaining treatment from a primary care physician could be, for all anyone knows, getting a flu shot. Ideally, seeing a psychiatrist would not be stigmatizing. But that is not the society we live in today.

On the other hand, people with serious co-occurring mental health conditions or significant polysubstance use are less likely to fare well outside of specialized addiction treatment settings.[220] One approach is for primary care physicians to diagnose the severity of the opioid addiction and then decide whether the patient needs specialized care. If yes, the primary care physician would send the patient to the specialist. If no, then the primary care physician would proceed to treat the patient. Even if the primary care physician sends the patient to a specialist, the specialist and primary care physician should continue to share patient information and work together as a treatment team. There are many conditions related to drug use, such as HIV/AIDS or hepatitis C, for which the primary care physician can continue to provide treatment. Furthermore, once the patient has stabilized and made significant progress in the specialist setting, the treatment can be "stepped down" and the patient can return to the primary care physician's office for maintenance medication.

Regrettably, provider collaboration in addiction treatment is impeded by their misunderstanding of privacy laws.[221] In addiction treatment, two privacy laws reign supreme: the Health Insurance Portability and Accountability Act (HIPAA) and Title 42 of the Federal Code of Regulations Part 2 (42 CFR 2). HIPAA and 42 CFR 2 were created at different times for different purposes.

HIPAA, and its associated regulations, applies to all private health information and protects patient privacy but also ensures flexibility in treatment and health insurance services, as the word "portability" in the name implies. In contrast, 42 CFR 2 was written decades before HIPAA with the purpose of preventing potentially stigmatizing substance use and mental health information from reaching unintended eyes and ears. It does not apply to health information generally, singling out and adding an extra layer of protection to substance use information specifically.

As a result, HIPAA and 42 CFR 2 differ in the extent to which they allow health care providers to share information about patients for purposes of treatment collaboration and integration *before* the health care provider must get special consent from the patient. Special consent means extra paperwork and associated liability risks. For example, HIPAA allows health professionals to share patients' private health information without obtaining patients' consent when the purpose of sharing information is for referral, consultation, or coordination of services.[222,223] This rule applies to all health conditions *except* substance use disorders.

For substance use disorders, providers must follow privacy regulations in 42 CFR 2. As originally written, 42 CFR 2 required treatment providers to obtain specific written consent from patients prior to sharing health information with other treatment providers, only allowing for a few narrow exceptions, such as life-threatening emergencies. The patient had to complete a document specifically naming the health care practitioner who would receive the information, defining the type of information to be shared, and stating the dates during which information could be shared. Each time a new health care provider came into the picture, such as a new counselor or primary care physician, a new form would need to be created and signed by the patient.

One might wonder why consent forms would serve as any kind of barrier to begin with. Isn't it easy for a patient to complete and sign a form? The problem is not so much on the patient's side but more so on the provider's side, as each additional layer of paperwork is time-consuming, requiring staff resources. Furthermore, 42 CFR 2 applies to substance use–related health data only, rather than to other health conditions, making the former *appear* more legally risky to collect and share. As my interviews with health care providers reveal, physicians and counselors are very sensitive to potential liability risks, even if these risks are theoretically easy to overcome or very remote. Additionally, most electronic health record systems do not allow for data segmentation, meaning separation of substance use–related health data from other types of medical data. Data segmentation would allow providers to share some parts of the electronic health record while hiding other parts, such as substance use data. But without data segmentation in the electronic health record systems, providers may have difficulty sharing *any* health information so long as substance use–related health data is embedded within the medical record.[221]

In response to numerous complaints about the tedious consent process involved in treating substance use disorders, in 2017 the US Department of Health and Human Services amended 42 CFR 2 to allow patients to sign a general consent form in which patients can essentially say to their provider, "I allow you to share my health information with any current or future treatment provider for treatment purposes," thereby eliminating the need for new consent forms each time a new provider becomes involved.[224] But existing evidence suggests that this change is largely unknown or misunderstood among treatment providers, who still think they need new consent forms for each new provider.[221]

Dr. Dennis Watson at the University of Illinois at Chicago has seen firsthand how both treatment services and research can be derailed by misunderstanding 42 CFR 2. In one of his projects, which involves connecting people in the emergency department who recently overdosed with peer support specialists, different floors of the same hospital are sometimes reluctant to share patient information. He says the health care providers often assume there are legal problems with information sharing even when there are none. The barriers can be even more extreme when communication involves parties from outside institutions, such as community health clinics trying to obtain data about hospital patients. Ultimately, it is the patient who suffers from this lack of coordination and integration.

Studies have demonstrated the feasibility and efficacy of starting recently overdosed patients in the emergency department on buprenorphine,[225,226] after which the patients are immediately transferred to a low-barrier buprenorphine treatment provider. Such short-term (up to seventy-two hours) buprenorphine provision without a DATA waiver is legally permissible.[227] But the buprenorphine treatment will automatically end in the hospital if the hospital and local treatment providers are hesitant to share patients' private health information, missing a potentially huge opportunity to prevent overdose reoccurrence.

Surprisingly little is known about whether the extra layer of privacy afforded by 42 CFR 2 actually encourages patients to seek treatment. Based on conversations with numerous people in recovery who have never even heard of HIPAA, I find it even less likely that most people in recovery have heard of 42 CFR 2. That begs the question why the regulation exists to begin with. If its purpose is to make people feel comfortable seeking treatment but most people are unaware of it, then are the regulations helping people seek treatment or are they merely deterring provider collaboration and integration? As one scholar has written, "The [42 CFR 2] regulations predate the creation of electronic health records and reflect a time when individuals with alcohol and drug use disorders were treated almost exclusively in stand-alone, specialized facilities."[221] In a different era when federal and state governments are pushing for greater integration of care, maybe it is time to heavily revise 42 CFR 2 or even eliminate it entirely, relying on HIPAA instead.

STIGMA TOWARD PEOPLE with addiction is pervasive, not just among the general public, but even among health care professionals. It adds yet another layer of barriers to the mountain of barriers to accessing addiction treatment. Although the American Medical Association has called addiction a disease for decades, some physicians are biased against people with addiction, mirroring the American public's biases. According to one survey, medical students frequently viewed addiction as a personal choice evolving from enjoyment, ignorance, or apathy; these misconceptions prompted medical school students to feel anger toward those who continue to harm themselves with drugs.[205] As one medical student wrote, "I think it will be difficult to deal with people who don't want to take an active role in improving their health." These misconceptions at best translate into poor physician-patient interactions, and at worst they will produce stunted professionals. According to the study, "[Medical students] did not appear to react as physicians when confronted with addiction patients. They did not discuss clinical features, diagnosis, medical treatment, or advice. . . . They did not convey a sense of therapeutic optimism and pride in their acquisition of clinical skills needed to help addicted patients."[205]

Such biases persist among practicing physicians. Addiction's nature as a relapsing condition can be especially frustrating for physicians who want to manage it but lack the appropriate tools or training. Other chronic relapsing conditions that physicians treat routinely, such as hypertension, carry less stigma, and physicians receive comprehensive training in their management. As Dr. Andrews, a primary care physician, explained, it becomes easy for the physician to give up, thinking, "Well, those people have weak personalities, or their upbringing wasn't good." Treatment failures are easier to excuse if addiction is framed as a personality issue and not a medical condition.

Moreover, physicians may also worry that patients with addiction will monopolize appointments, changing clinic environments and driving other patients to new providers.[178] According to one psychiatrist, "I think the fear is, if I open the door a crack, it's going to be overwhelming. My office staff is going to be inundated with all these addicts with their needles and their waiting. This, I think, is a fanciful fear. What I want to tell them is a good twenty percent, thirty percent, even forty percent of your patients are already struggling with addiction and have not told you." Indeed, a recent study found that the main reason physicians do not seek a DATA waiver is "not wanting to be inundated with requests for buprenorphine."[228] Physicians may also worry that the stigma surrounding addiction will rub off on themselves. As Dr. Cohen explained, "Stigma rubs off and so if you're a patient with a psychiatry disorder there is still a stigma associated with that. There's even more with people who are addicted, if you can believe it. The people who treat them are seen as kind of the dregs of medical practice."

Relatedly, much research suggests physicians rarely want to treat patients with addiction because they are supposedly "difficult" and act in undesirable and antisocial ways, such as being manipulative and dishonest.[178,229] My research suggests that the fear of "difficult" patients may be related to lack of training. Unlike physicians with little experience treating addiction, physicians trained in addiction medicine are often quick to point out that "difficult" patients become great patients once the disease is managed. In fact, treating addiction often turns into one of the most rewarding experiences of the physician's career. The physician witnesses the patient's entire life turned around: from finding a job, to rekindling relationships with significant others and family members, to leaving the revolving door of the criminal justice system.

Physicians must learn that difficult behaviors associated with addiction are really symptoms of the medical condition, but this learning process requires empathy for patients, meaning a willingness to put oneself in patients' shoes and to imagine how patients experience the world. Empathy is critical to treatment relationships and enhances treatment success. Contact and interaction with a stigmatized population increases empathy for the population; so, increasing medical students' and residents' interactions with patients who have addiction may increase empathy for this vulnerable group. Professional empathy training also may help physicians understand why patients with addiction act out, learn not to take such actions personally, and acquire skills to manage them. Though understudied, empathy training may take place in small groups of physicians who debrief after patient meetings to discuss what happened and why. Improved communication skills training could also improve physicians' interactions with patients, easing potential confrontation and anger toward patients. Patients confronted with an annoyed or hostile physician may feel mistreated and stigmatized, pulling back from the relationship, possibly never seeking addiction treatment again.

Even physicians who want to treat patients with addiction may find that their institutions or coworkers would prefer to refer these patients out. In one study, as many as 42 percent of primary care physicians cited resistance from practice partners and 36 percent named institutional resistance as barriers to buprenorphine treatment.[230] Such resistance may stem from common misconceptions about addiction and MAT. For example, if institutions or coworkers view buprenorphine as "just another drug," then physicians prescribing buprenorphine are seen as "enablers."

Such myths are reinforced by the perception that buprenorphine is widely misused or abused. In fact, some people do purchase buprenorphine illicitly on the street or over the internet, but they typically do so to prevent withdrawal symptoms.[61,72,231–233] The government reports that when people with opioid addiction experience opioid withdrawal symptoms, the symptoms are typically so strong that they return to using opioids.[234] For heroin users, withdrawal symptoms may appear as soon as four hours since their last heroin use.[180] Buprenorphine can help fill that gap. For example, when I ask Stan, who has a history of illicit buprenorphine purchases, why he and others have bought buprenorphine on the street, he responds, "It's definitely about preventing withdrawal. It's usually people who are like, oh, I'm going to get clean. And so they put aside ten dollars each day or whatever it is, and they find themselves, seven days' worth of strips. A lot of times these people fail because they don't have the surrounding support. But I've had friends who have done it."

Street buprenorphine purchases can also bridge people into formal treatment, assuming they can find a provider and pay. Some people do purchase buprenorphine illicitly to get high but that is exaggerated, especially by criminal justice administrators. As Stan further explained about buprenorphine, "It's a miserable [high]! There's a joke kind of street name called subaaaaaaaaahxone—like a puking noise—because if you take it and you don't need it, it'll make you really ill and it will make you throw up. It's a really unpleasant high. Like if you take enough of it for yourself to feel something, you're usually also going to feel really nauseous . . . get headaches . . . feel unpleasantly warm." Nevertheless, misunderstandings about illicit buprenorphine use may prompt providers or their institutions to avoid prescribing it, especially if they fear that it may cause a liability risk.

Some institutional characteristics significantly influence whether a clinic is likely to adopt MAT. For example, clinics that are more likely to adopt MAT are accredited, are hospital-affiliated, provide inpatient care, and/or provide detoxification services.[235,236] In contrast, institutions promoting abstinence-only treatment are particularly resistant to adopting MAT,[150] as are institutions that lack affiliations with hospitals or other medical practices, perhaps due to lower physician involvement in addiction treatment and separation from mainstream medicine in general.

Changing attitudes within a health care institution takes time. For institutional changes to trickle down from the top levels of health care bureaucracies, employees in lower levels of bureaucracies must be exposed to the new practice, perceive a need to change existing practices, decide to adopt the new practice because it is demonstrably useful, and begin using the new practice. This process may take years from start to finish.

Sometimes institutional change begins not at the top but at the bottom, from providers. Dr. Miller works for a large addiction and mental health treatment organization serving hundreds of patients with opioid addiction. Just three years ago, the organization was a classic abstinence-only institution that explicitly barred clients undergoing MAT from participating in group counseling or support groups on the premises. As a former employee of both a methadone clinic and an office-based buprenorphine treatment practice, Dr. Miller brought extensive addiction treatment experience with her into her new work environment. Despite having no formal leadership role, within a few years Dr. Miller had dramatically changed institutional beliefs about MAT, partially through organizing educational MAT seminars for all staff members, including counselors, physicians, and administrators, and partially from one-on-one conversations with resistant administrators. It was not long before she received administrative permission to provide MAT, becoming the first physician in the practice to prescribe buprenorphine and extended-release naltrexone.

According to Dr. Miller, colleagues' and administrators' acceptance of MAT grew after they saw positive treatment results. Yet a lingering resistance to MAT still exists, particularly from peer support specialists, who are often in recovery themselves through abstinence-only methods. Sometimes they misinform patients, telling them to wean off MAT as quickly as possible, contrary to best medical practices. Thus, Dr. Miller must continually remind colleagues that long-term use of MAT is more effective than short-term use. In her ongoing attempt to change institutional culture and practices, she stresses the importance of providing regular, ongoing education about MAT to all staff members. High workforce turnover rates also necessitate such repeated educational efforts.

Finally, institutional cultural change can be coerced. Large public treatment centers frequently receive at least some, if not most, of their funding from federal, state, or local governments. This gives the government carrots and sticks to persuade treatment centers to adopt evidence-based policies. Not surprisingly, one national study found that when state mental health authorities made public funding of addiction treatment centers contingent on allowing MAT, MAT implementation increased.[237]

SUPPOSE THAT A PHYSICIAN has a DATA waiver and works in an institution supportive of addiction treatment, including MAT. Further suppose that this physician has adequate addiction medicine education and empathy for patients with addiction. Surely this physician will be willing to prescribe medications for treating addiction, such as buprenorphine or extended-release naltrexone, right? Unfortunately, other layers of barriers may still remain. One of the most common is insurance restrictions.

Before 2008, insurance companies often made it harder for patients to access treatment for mental health and addiction than treatment for other chronic health conditions. Such disparities prompted Congress to pass the Mental Health Parity and Addiction Equity Act of 2008, which prohibits differences in treatment limits, cost sharing, and in-network/out-of-network coverage between treatment for physical illness and treatment for mental health or addiction. A few years later, the Affordable Care Act broadened the Mental Health Parity and Addiction Equity Act so that it now applies to Medicaid-managed care organizations, the Children's Health Insurance Program, small and large employer-funded plans, commercial health insurance sold on the Affordable Care Act marketplace, and Medicaid

Alternative Benefit Plans.[238] Furthermore, the Affordable Care Act required most health insurance plans to cover treatment for mental health disorders and addiction as an essential health benefit.[238]

But it is increasingly clear that the Mental Health Parity and Addiction Equity Act has not truly created parity for mental health and addiction treatment. Many health insurers continue to place onerous burdens on people seeking treatment for these conditions. Burdens on patients translate into burdens on physicians who try to help patients get treatment covered. The physicians I have interviewed overwhelmingly agree that parity does not exist. Some responses have been tinged with anger, such as Dr. Curry's response: "Oh, is there supposed to be parity? I've never seen it!" At addiction-themed conferences, providers openly air their grievances about insurance burdens, including how insurance companies waste their time and staff time with unnecessary paperwork, preventing them from caring for patients. The highest level of anger is directed toward insurance prior authorization requirements.

Completing a prior authorization form may sound simple, but it is actually very time-consuming, with separate forms required for each patient on MAT. One study of DATA-waivered physicians who accept Medicaid found that prior authorizations were the highest rated barrier to prescribing buprenorphine.[239] Furthermore, prior authorization requirements for buprenorphine may increase relapse rates, at least in the short-term.[240] Dr. Lopez described how his office had to hire an additional billing specialist just to complete preauthorizations and argue with insurance companies that denied coverage. Other physicians decided to stop prescribing altogether. Unfortunately, prior authorization requirements are widespread. A 2015 study found that 94 percent of state Medicaid programs require prior authorization for MAT,[241] and a 2016 study found that 85 percent of private insurance plans nationwide require prior authorization for extended-release naltrexone.[242] But recently some states, such as California[243] and Pennsylvania,[244] have begun removing prior authorization requirements from their Medicaid programs in response to the escalating opioid overdose crisis.

If seeking prior authorizations weren't bad enough, additional insurance rules compound this burden for physicians. Since addiction is a chronic medical condition, physicians must regularly renew each patient's MAT prior authorizations—and insurers don't necessarily accept renewals until the previous prior authorization has expired, preventing physicians from submitting prior authorization forms ahead of time. These delays in accessing treatment can be deadly. If a prior authorization expires on January 1 and a patient runs out of buprenorphine that day, she might not be able to receive a prescription by January 3 unless the prior authorization is submitted immediately. Buprenorphine only remains in a patient's system for two to three days before the patient begins undergoing withdrawal and cravings return, putting the patient at serious risk of relapse and overdose.

Additionally, when completing prior authorization forms for buprenorphine, physicians are sometimes required to tell an insurance company how soon they plan to wean the patient off MAT. Some insurers require physicians to promise in writing to wean the patient off after only six months or one year. But medical studies conclude that long-term, not short-term, buprenorphine treatment is more effective.[240,245] Arbitrary treatment termination deadlines also increase relapse rates.[245] In response, some physicians tell insurance companies they will wean patients off MAT without actually intending to do so, or they attach a note describing their displeasure with the insurance requirement. After the six-month or one-year period has elapsed, the physicians must once again participate in the prior authorization process. According to some physicians I have interviewed, insurers rarely require provider promises to wean patients off of other medications, including prescription painkillers such as oxycodone. Therefore, these "weaning" requirements appear to violate federal parity law.

Insurance providers also have other arbitrary rules about what they will and will not pay for. Multiple physicians have reported that their state Medicaid program won't pay for extended-release naltrexone stored in physicians' offices. Instead patients must first attend a physician appointment to receive a diagnosis and a written prescription for extended-release naltrexone; next, the patient must go to a pharmacy to pick up the medication or have it mailed from a specialty pharmacy, which can take days; finally, the patient must return once more to the physician's office to have the medication administered for the first time, called "induction."

For extended-release naltrexone patients, induction requires that the health care provider inject the medication into the patient, potentially followed by a two- to four-hour observation period. Unfortunately, patients who are required to leave the physician's office to visit a pharmacy or wait for a mail delivery before induction may never make it to the pharmacy or back to the physician. Even a simple trigger, such as seeing a building where the patient has previously gotten high, may overwhelm his or her motivation. Addiction often gives patients only a short and critical window of time during which they are willing and able to undergo treatment. If that window disappears, it may be a long time until a new window appears, and in the meantime, the patient risks overdosing.

As if arbitrary and unfair insurance rules weren't enough, low addiction treatment reimbursement rates may further deter physicians, especially within Medicaid programs.[228] Medicaid covers most addiction treatment in the United States, since addiction is associated with lower incomes.[246] But Medicaid reimbursement rates for physicians are significantly lower than commercial health insurance rates and Medicare rates.[247] Even commercial health insurers often reimburse addiction treatment at lower rates than other covered procedures.[248] Addiction treatment appointments do not involve expensive surgical procedures or machines; instead, they rely on physician-patient counseling, monitoring, and medication prescribing. None of these procedures garner high reimbursement rates to begin with, a problem that plagues behavioral health care in general.

Low reimbursement rates for addiction treatment, especially in Medicaid programs, are not inevitable. They reflect a government policy choice and the stigmatization of behavioral health care and low-income people in general. In France, in contrast, physicians are paid more by the government for management of chronic diseases than treatment of other diseases, and addiction is considered a chronic disease.[64] Higher physician reimbursement for addiction treatment helps counteract existing stigma toward patients with addiction.

Many Americans fall in an insurance gap in which they are ineligible for Medicaid because they make too much money for the program that targets the truly indigent, but they lack commercial insurance through an employer and cannot afford insurance on the individual market, which can be very expensive. Classic examples of people who fall in this gap include part-time employees, such as restaurant servers, or individuals who work full-time for small businesses that cannot afford to provide health insurance to their employees. For these Americans to afford addiction treatment and for physicians and treatment centers to accept them, government block grants are critical.[249] Such grants are particularly important in states that refused to expand Medicaid, thereby often leaving single, childless men ineligible for the insurance. Grants enable health care institutions to accept patients without health insurance on a sliding scale of payments depending on their income. One study found that such block grant funding for MAT was associated with more DATA-waivered physicians.[219] Whether from the state or federal government, such grants offer an opportunity to promote best practices if required under the grant.

Encouraging more physicians to treat addiction will depend on how Congress and state legislatures react to insurance-imposed barriers to addiction treatment and whether they increase reimbursement rates for behavioral health care. Government agencies should regularly assess insurance barriers to mental health and addiction treatment. Insurers whose policies violate federal parity laws should face severe consequences. Currently, enforcement of federal parity laws occurs in a piecemeal, uncoordinated manner, and patients and health care providers may not know whom to turn to when facing discrimination from insurers. For example, typically state insurance commissioners enforce federal parity laws for insurance plans with less than fifty-one employees; the Department of Labor and the Internal Revenue Service share enforcement authority for plans subject to the Employee Retirement Income Security Act; and the Department of Health and Human Services enforces self-funded, nongovernmental plans, as well as some small group plans. Such patchwork enforcement should be simplified. How is the patient or health care provider to know whom to contact in the event of a parity law violation?

AS FRUSTRATING AS INSURANCE barriers are for physicians, they harm patients more directly, sometimes leading them to cease addiction treatment altogether or to engage in sketchy system workarounds, such as illicit street purchases. When insurance coverage is inadequate, patients with limited means must decide whether to purchase medical care or food, or even whether they should sell some of their medication to afford the remainder of their treatment.

In early 2017, Brianna began work as a cashier at a gas station in a Midwestern city. It was the first stable job she had had in a long time. She is very proud of her progress, having already advanced from cashier to assistant manager when I interviewed her in the spring of 2018. She has not missed a single day of work nor has she ever arrived late. But the slight increase in her paycheck associated with her new position as assistant manager has made her ineligible for food stamps and her state's Medicaid program. Brianna doesn't really mind losing the food stamps because she can mostly afford her groceries these days, but the loss of Medicaid has hit her very hard. She is paying for commercial insurance, but the deductible is $3,000, a nearly impossible amount for her to afford. After starting her new insurance plan, she went to the pharmacy to pick up the buprenorphine prescription for which she had previously only paid $20 per month. She learned she must now pay $300 per month until she meets the deductible. Since she couldn't afford the entire month's supply, she asked for a five-day supply instead until she could figure out what to do.

Currently Brianna has a prescription for two daily strips of a buprenorphine, but she rarely takes the full daily dose. "Right now, I'm doing everything I can to just to stay on it, and there are days that I'll do one or one and a half [strips] or just try to keep them, so that way I don't run out, and I don't have to go without. I will take less, so that way I can make it last a little bit longer." Unfortunately, taking too low of a dose is risky. It can lead to withdrawal symptoms, and cravings can reemerge. Brianna explains, "There's days that I have to take two because I don't know if my body can take it. I don't feel good." She had quit the medication entirely once before, did fine for a while, but ultimately relapsed. Now she's determined to continue the treatment no matter what. Brianna's even considered going to the emergency room, just to rack up a high enough bill at the hospital that it would cover her deductible. Then she could get on a hospital income-based repayment plan. Unfortunately, she explains, she doesn't have any condition that would qualify as an emergency.

LIKE BRIANNA, ANDY BEGAN Suboxone treatment for his oxycodone addiction while in the Midwest. He believes Suboxone saved his life, completely stopping his misuse of opioids. Over three years, he decreased his Suboxone dose from 16 mg daily to 2 mg daily. Though he no longer had cravings at the 2 mg dose, he decided he still wanted MAT, just in case. He thought Vivitrol would be a great option. He was tired of taking the Suboxone film every morning, and he wasn't going to miss the nausea that sometimes came with it. He also wasn't going to miss the strange looks he regularly received from the local

CVS pharmacist, whose attitude toward him always dipped after seeing the medication name on the prescription paper. And no other CVS in the city carried Suboxone.

He decided to switch to Vivitrol as he was moving across the country for a new job. Now located in a large metropolis, he thought finding a Vivitrol provider would be easy, but in some ways it proved more difficult than starting Suboxone. First, he needed to undergo inpatient detoxification. He was terrified of undergoing detoxification outside of a treatment center, even from the low dose of Suboxone, after having read horror stories on the internet of painful experiences from people who tried to detoxify alone at home. But Andy's commercial insurance only covered inpatient detoxification for alcohol addiction, not opioid addiction. Detoxification from alcohol is potentially deadly, since some people get life-threatening seizures, while detoxification from opioids is not itself deadly even though relapse, of course, can be. Not giving up, he tried a different tactic. Since he had noticed that he'd been drinking too much lately, he asked the insurance company to pay for alcohol detoxification with the co-occurring condition of opioid addiction. Now his insurance was willing to pay, though it left Andy with a coinsurance bill of almost $1,000, something he is still paying off.

Even though detoxification was a necessary step to beginning Vivitrol, the detoxification center did not actually offer Vivitrol. In fact, it offered nothing at all, except group counseling and on-site AA meetings while monitoring him and providing palliative care. With detoxification completed, he began the hunt for an outpatient Vivitrol provider. According to an internet search, about a dozen existed in his city, but by calling them he learned that most either only accepted cash payments or were not accepting new patients. Finally, he found an outpatient clinic that treated addiction and claimed to offer Vivitrol. What it actually offered, though, was an intake appointment, at which a counselor asked a series of questions meant to determine whether Vivitrol might be an appropriate medication.

Determining this to be the case, the counselor then passed Andy off to a psychiatrist in a different office—an appointment that was not available until two months later. Andy met with the psychiatrist, who prescribed Vivitrol but still did not actually provide the medication. Instead, the psychiatrist sent Andy's information to a special-order pharmacy, as per insurance requirements, which then mailed the medication directly to a third location—where the medication would finally be administered by nurses. But the third location, a "home infusion center" did not have any openings for another month. In total, by the time Andy received his first Vivitrol injection, over four months had passed since detoxification. Fortunately, Andy was stable and did not relapse, but he is deeply concerned about others less stable than him going through this process. He is almost certain that they would not make it.

6

WHEN CRIMINAL JUSTICE ADMINISTRATORS MAKE MEDICAL DECISIONS

CANDACE SAYS HER RECOVERY STORY "isn't linear." I tell her that is okay and, as far as I can tell, really common. In other words, she has been in recovery for years but has had periods of relapse, which are becoming less and less frequent over time. If she compares her life today to her life ten years ago, there is no doubt that she is doing better.

Candace started using opiates when she was eighteen, but that was not her first drug—just her favorite drug, and the one she couldn't stop no matter how hard she tried. She remembers first wanting to use drugs in the second grade. Her parents had been watching the nightly news, and the news anchor described children sniffing glue in class to get high. The next day, Candace tried it. She tells me over the phone, "I wonder if maybe I was just kind of born a little bit unbalanced." As a baby, she used to self-harm, which she believes was an indicator of future depression. In fact, throughout her life Candace has had extreme bouts of depression, including suicide attempts. She suspects that drugs may have initially served as a coping mechanism, but even after receiving treatment for depression, the cravings for drugs continued.

At twenty years old, feeling depressed and ashamed that her life's purpose now consisted of obtaining and using heroin, she began an intensive outpatient program. The IOP she joined consisted of almost daily group counseling and biweekly individual counseling. Despite regular attendance, however, she still spent all day thinking about getting high. The cravings were too intense for the IOP alone to help. She wanted additional help and knew residential rehab wouldn't cut it. Her parents had once paid for an expensive rehab in the Northeast, consisting entirely of detoxification, twelve-step programming, and counseling; as soon as she left, she had relapsed.

Candace decided to enroll in formal Suboxone treatment, hoping to add it to her IOP regimen. She had previously bought Suboxone on the street to prevent withdrawal symptoms, and she remembered it had helped with cravings too. Additionally, she had once tried heroin shortly after taking Suboxone and the combination made her violently sick. No longer wanting to buy medications off the street, she asked the IOP if they offered Suboxone. They said no. And furthermore, they said if they found out she was utilizing Suboxone, she would not be able to participate in some of the group counseling.

Fortunately, another former drug user suggested that Candace contact a new buprenorphine provider that had just opened a clinic across town. The clinic provided two things: weekly group counseling and weekly buprenorphine prescriptions. The clinic required participation in both treatment modalities simultaneously. Candace was not excited about resuming group counseling. She remembers walking in one day at the IOP with her hair disheveled and clothes unwashed but proud of herself for showing up despite cravings and feeling sick. Seeing how Candace looked, however, the counselor suggested that she put more work into her appearance. Since then, group counseling had always felt awkward. The main reason Candace continued at all was that group counseling at the IOP was a corequisite of individual counseling—in other words, you couldn't attend individual counseling if you weren't also attending group counseling. And Candace really liked her individual counselor who helped her work through some of her mental health issues.

When Candace began regular buprenorphine treatment across town, she was surprised to find the group counseling more helpful than it had been at the IOP. It occurred much less frequently—just for one hour, once per week—but in some ways it felt more relevant. Much of the discussion explicitly addressed medication compliance, side effects, and stigma surrounding buprenorphine. It was not twelve-step based, though some patients did attend Alcoholics Anonymous or Narcotics Anonymous in the community too.

For one year, Candace made significant progress. Her parents were speaking to her again, and she even started working on a bachelor's degree at the local university. Unfortunately, since starting her on the buprenorphine program, the providers had repeatedly told her that buprenorphine was not intended to be used long term and that the clinic policy required tapering after one year. Exceptions were sometimes granted; but, perversely, they were never granted to people who had fully stabilized and appeared to be doing well—even if medication was the reason they were doing well. As expected, after about one year, the provider tapered Candace off. Even though while on a stable dose she could go days without thinking about getting high, the tapering process terrified her. It felt too fast, and her old cravings began to reemerge. But clinic policy was strict: no long-term buprenorphine treatment. About two months after quitting the lowest dose of buprenorphine, she started using again.

After once again feeling her life spiral out of control, Candace called the buprenorphine clinic, explaining that she had relapsed. The clinic said she could restart treatment. As before, she resumed weekly group meetings and weekly buprenorphine prescriptions, which she took at home daily. About one year later, the clinic tapered her off again, as per clinic policy. As before, she was fine for a few weeks without the medication and then relapsed.

PRESSURE FOR CANDACE TO QUIT buprenorphine has not only come from her prescriber. It has also come from the criminal justice system. In fact, Candace's worst relapse occurred while she was participating in a local drug court program. As she describes her experience over the phone, she breaks into tears. We pause the interview multiple times, but Candace is adamant about sharing her story in case it helps others.

The second time the clinic forced Candace to taper off buprenorphine, she returned to heroin use. One day, the cops pulled her over for driving erratically, immediately noticing that she was high. They searched the car and found an empty syringe with trace amounts of heroin. She did not try to argue, accepting her fate as they booked her into the city jail. Then a miracle seemingly occurred—she was given the opportunity to participate in the local drug court rather than face imprisonment.

Drug courts are special courts, called problem-solving courts, where the goal is not merely punishment but also rehabilitation. In theory, the judge and his or her "treatment team" assist you on your recovery journey, becoming almost like a second family. In fact, some drug court judges take on parental roles, asking participants about their personal relationships, progress with employment, and feelings as well as providing advice in these highly personal areas. It is a strange hat for a presumably neutral, unbiased decision-maker to wear.

Currently, over three thousand drug courts exist in the United States.[250] To a certain extent, each drug court is unique, with its own policies, priorities, and biases—an island in the criminal justice system. Nevertheless, there are certain practices you can expect to see in most: regular hearings in front of a judge and your fellow participants wherein your recent successes or failures are publicly discussed; random urine drug screens; closed treatment-team staff meetings wherein treatment requirements and participation are discussed; case manager–participant meetings; and, of course, treatment. In my study of Indiana[104] and Florida drug courts, I have rarely seen courts provide treatment, though Florida courts sometimes pay for it. Rather, treatment usually occurs at an affiliated outside clinic but is carefully monitored by the court treatment team. Often, one of the counselors or case managers on the court staff works at a large treatment agency, making information sharing seamless.[104,251]

Despite being called a "treatment team," the drug court staff is really supposed to be there to monitor or enforce treatment, with treatment decisions made by qualified health care providers, such as nurse practitioners or physicians. Hardly any of the treatment team members have a medical background, with the team typically consisting of a judge (the team head), attorneys, law enforcement, the prosecutor, case managers, court administrators, and a sprinkling of counselors.[104,252] Counselors may or may not have graduate degrees. In my 2016–2017 study of twenty Indiana drug courts and veterans' courts (which are like drug courts but for veterans), only two teams included a physician.

One may wonder how a court treatment team with essentially no medical personnel led by a judge can properly assist participants in recovery, especially with respect to medication-assisted treatment. I certainly did. According to governmental agencies, judges and their staff are *supposed* to rely on medication decisions of qualified health care practitioners, with the nonclinical team members enforcing the clinicians' decisions through predictable, graduated sanctions.[252] But in my interviews with judges in courts from two states, Indiana and Florida, I have found wide discrepancies with this preferred approach. Some drug court judges enforce the decision made by clinicians without second-guessing clinicians' motivation or effectiveness, while other judges seem to treat clinicians' decisions as nothing more than a recommendation that can be discarded if it fails to fit into the abstinence-only philosophy of the court treatment team. As a result, people with opioid use disorders who should have access to MAT are often prohibited from having potentially lifesaving medication.

I ASK CANDACE TO DESCRIBE her experience in drug court, and her experience is not dissimilar from the experiences of some others whom I have interviewed. When provided the opportunity of drug court rather than incarceration, Candace felt she had been granted a gift—the opportunity to clear her criminal record, so long as she completed all the drug court requirements, including treatment, successfully.

She entered drug court full steam ahead. She attended the mandatory hearings, took the random urine drug screens, went to the required group counseling at the same IOP center she had once attended, and participated almost daily in AA. Very quickly, however, she knew she needed medication too. To her knowledge, no official court policy prohibited Suboxone treatment, but she asked her case manager just in case. The case manager asked the judge, who discussed the idea with the court treatment team. The treatment team said no.

I ask Candace whether she was surprised by the treatment team's response. She wasn't. Explaining herself, Candace described the following story. During one court hearing, in which all court participants stand as a group in front of the judge and answer the judge's questions, a fellow participant casually mentioned that some people get high off gabapentin, a nonopioid medication for nerve pain. Hearing the comment, the judge turned to another participant and said, "Hey, aren't you on that stuff?" The participant nodded, to which the judge responded, "Oh, you're not anymore, honey." The participant had been taking gabapentin to prevent seizures and a short time later suffered one.

Reflecting on the judge's role on the treatment team, Candace says, "[Judges] are deciding what treatment you get and how you are treated very literally, and they have no training for it . . . and there wasn't a doctor on staff saying this medication is okay for this person." I ask whom the judge was receiving medical advice from. Candace says, "He was getting his advice from counselors, but our head counselor had gone to school at the University of Phoenix, and it was just for counseling. It's not the same as a doctor." I ask why no physicians participated on the treatment team. Candace thinks it's because they are too expensive and the court can't afford them.

This reason rings true. In a series of interviews with drug court judges, I repeatedly heard that paying for additional staff is virtually impossible. In fact, drug court staff often hold multiple roles in the criminal justice system to keep court costs down, with funding for one role subsidizing the other role. For example, a full-time felony court judge will become a drug court judge one day per week, with the salary for the drug court role paid by the felony court position. It's the same deal with probation officers, law enforcement, prosecutors, and multiple other treatment team members, many of whom wear a drug court staff member "hat" one day per week. Paying for a physician would require extra money that in many tightly stretched counties simply does not exist. And frankly, it is not clear to me that many physicians would be interested in the job, even for a few hours per week. Physician interviews have revealed that they often don't take kindly to the idea of having their medical decisions or expertise potentially overruled by a judge with no medical training. In fact, a 2019 ethics bulletin from the American Society of Addiction Medicine urges physicians to maintain autonomy in decision-making as far as possible, even when criminal justice system employees try to impose their own views regarding treatment.[253]

Candace's time in drug court proved heartbreaking. Unable to access the only treatment that she felt had ever helped, she repeatedly relapsed. Even though the first few relapses resulted in little more than a slap on the wrist, with punishments ranging from more AA meetings to writing an essay about the dangers of drug use, the sanctions eventually became more and more severe. She remembers once being given a week in jail, which proved particularly unfortunate given that she was in the middle of pursuing her bachelor's degree. Interestingly, the court team decided to spread out the jail time to let Candace continue attending university classes during the weekdays, but in exchange she had to spend each weekend of an entire month in jail. Unfortunately, Candace continued relapsing, always to heroin. Finally, the judge had had enough. Candace was ousted from the court program and incarcerated for a few months. She was unable to finish her bachelor's degree while in jail and no longer has the heart to start it again.

Today, Candace is on probation and on her third stint at the buprenorphine clinic. Unfortunately, she feels like the only way to stay at the clinic long-term is to repeatedly relapse, with no reward for doing well on a stable dose. Candace says some people from the clinic have done just fine after the taper, but she is not one of those people. She explains, "I guess that's kind of how the pattern has been for most of my life without maintenance treatments; I usually last about three months. The maintenance doesn't have to be opiates. I've also done Vivitrol, and I do really well on that too." Unfortunately, Vivitrol is even less accessible in her city than buprenorphine and is very costly.

I ask her why the buprenorphine clinic insists on tapering her off. She responds, "The goal is for nothing [meaning, no medication], which now when I look at it, that's really weird to me, because I see family members who take lithium and the doctors are in no hurry. And it's the same for so many other medications that people take; there's not this inherent desire to get them off. So now I see it as weird; but at the time, I just thought, of course that's the goal."

She thinks insurance providers also exert some of the pressure; she remembers a prescribing doctor at the clinic saying tapering looks good for insurance purposes. As I speak to her, I can hear the tension in her voice. I ask if she is worried about having to come off Suboxone again. She answers, "Oh yeah, but it's something I'd just rather not think about."

IN 2017, CURTIS HILL, the Republican attorney general of Indiana publicly stated that incarceration is good for drug users, helping them jump-start recovery. In fact, he called longer jail terms more "compassionate" than shorter jail terms.[254] His argument rested on two highly questionable assumptions: first, that quality treatment is available in jails; and two, that jails give people an "Aha!" moment, motivating them to start treatment. In some ways, the arguments resemble those from the Anslinger era and those voiced by Nelson Rockefeller, the adamant supporter of mandatory minimum drug sentences.

One could examine the attorney general's statement from a number of angles and arrive at the same conclusion—that he is wrong, and that sticking people in jail or prison for drug use or possession is actually impractical and harmful. From a fiscal standpoint alone, it doesn't seem to make sense. An often-cited study in California found that every dollar spent on addiction treatment saves four dollars in health care costs and seven dollars on law enforcement costs.[255] Addiction treatment in the community more than pays for itself, particularly by helping people avoid incarceration. Additionally, incarceration is a failed strategy for preventing relapse. One study estimates that 95 percent of inmates incarcerated for drug offenses will resume substance use within three years of release, with one-third resuming substance use in only two months.[256]

I decided to examine the effect of incarceration on recovery by interviewing people in recovery—particularly those who had experienced addiction treatment, or the lack thereof, in the criminal justice system. During in-depth confidential phone interviews with people in recovery, about half of whom came from Indiana, I repeated the attorney general's claim and asked if they had any comment on the matter. Did they agree or disagree, or were they unsure? Almost four dozen people answered the question. Not one person agreed with Hill's statement and the vast majority believed that putting someone with an addiction in jail or prison actually causes the opposite result—relapse, or at least a delay in the recovery process.

I accumulated so many powerful, memorable quotes in response to this question, that it took me some time to decide which ones to include in this book. Even interviewees who had until that point been entirely matter-of-fact and unemotional in their interview responses suddenly turned passionate after hearing Hill's claim. They did not hesitate in giving clear explanations for why jail or prison was bad for recovery. The financial impact, for one, can be enormous, costing one's employment and saddling one with debt. Poverty is not a great foundation for recovery. As one of my favorite addiction psychiatrists in Indiana explained, you have to have something to live for! If you are homeless and unemployed, recovery may not even seem worth it; the warm feeling of drugs running through your veins may be the closest you'll feel to happiness all day, so why give it up?

Relatedly, criminalization increases shame, something that people in recovery says makes you want to use drugs more, not less. According to Sarah, "When you're in the depths of that sickness and that dark place, you don't like yourself and you're already shaming yourself." In response to throwing someone in jail or prison for using, Sarah says, "You talk about shame and stigma and reasons to keep using? That's another reason to keep using. And another reason to hate yourself." Multiple people argued that criminalizing the symptoms of a disorder is counterintuitive to treating the disorder. Alyssa thinks it's hypocritical to put anyone in jail or prison who committed a drug-related crime due to a health condition. She says even television anchors are calling addiction a disease these days: "It just seems like we don't believe what we're publishing [in the medical literature]."

One of the strongest arguments against jail or prison for drug use is that it can disrupt a recovery process that has already started, keeping in mind that recovery is rarely a onetime, relapse-free experience but is more often experienced as a journey with fewer and fewer relapses, hopefully resulting in an end to dangerous drug use all together. James, who is in recovery himself and helps direct a syringe exchange program on the East Coast, described helping connect Rick, a young man, to the local methadone clinic. They became acquainted when Rick joined the syringe exchange program and was still regularly using heroin. After just a few weeks at the methadone clinic, Rick had almost entirely stopped using heroin and was attending group counseling. Most importantly, he was motivated to stop drug use and felt that he had the tools to do so, given enough time. Then he got arrested for paraphernalia possession. Rick was thrown into jail by the local judge for forty-five days. According to James, before the jail time, Rick was stabilizing: "He'd started getting his stuff together in recovery." But in jail, Rick was forced to endure a painful, cold-turkey detoxification from methadone that disrupted everything. Frustrated, James explains, "Rick got out and now he's back in that cycle [of regular heroin use]. He just got incarcerated again the other day. It's just a mess." James is confident that if Rick had not been arrested, he would be further along in recovery than he is today.

And then, of course, there is the frequently voiced argument that jail and prison are rampant with drugs to begin with. As interviewees describe it, if you take people and throw them into a cage where they are miserable, the prison drug dealer becomes the most popular person—he or she is the only source of happiness experienced during the day. And while using drugs in prison, incarcerated people are actively thinking about how to access more drugs upon release. Even people in a high security prison, where hardly any drugs seep into the cells, often feel miserable enough that their first plan of action upon leaving is to get high. This may be one of the reasons that people leaving prison are at exponentially higher risk of overdose death than are nonincarcerated people.[257] Furthermore, people incarcerated for minor drug convictions are frequently mixed in jails and prisons with people convicted of violent crimes or other very serious violations. With plenty of time on their hands, incarcerated people learn from each other. Rather than being a time of rehabilitation, one interviewee stated, "Prison is graduate school for criminals."

Most directly addressing Hill's point, no interviewee stated that he or she obtained adequate treatment in jail or prison. This is not surprising in light of the published evidence. For example, fewer than 20 percent of incarcerated people have access to MAT,[258] even though a meta-analysis* of dozens of studies found that connecting people to MAT in prison or jail decreases opioid misuse and relapse, increasing postincarceration treatment engagement by a factor of seven, and through postincarceration treatment engagement may decrease re-incarceration rates and opioid overdoses.[259]

IT SEEMS CLEAR THAT JAIL or prison time is an impractical and damaging way to deal with opioid addiction. Are drug courts any better?

In 2016, I became fascinated with a particular question: What does treatment for opioid addiction look like in drug court? As someone trained in both law and public health, I found the intersection of the criminal justice system and medical world intriguing. I quickly discovered that very little information was published about treatment practices in drug courts. Legal scholars of drug courts referred to "treatment" in vague, generic terms in their publications without defining the type or efficacy of treatment provided.[260,261] Studies of treatment practices and policies for opioid addiction in drug courts were almost nonexistent. Yet effective treatment for opioid addiction in drug courts was and still is desperately needed. In a 2010 national study, approximately half of drug courts reported that 20 percent or more of their participants had opioid use disorder.[262] Rates have likely continued to rise.

Except for the groundbreaking 2010 study by Matusow et al. (published in 2013),[262] few studies have examined MAT access in

* Meta-analyses examine and pool results from many independent studies after excluding those with bad methodologies. Among analytic techniques for determining the evidence-base for medical treatments, meta-analysis is considered the top of the pyramid of approaches for weighing the efficacy of medical treatments. For more information, see "Meta-analysis: What, Why, and How" on the Cochrane UK website (https://uk.cochrane.org/news/meta-analysis-what-why-and-how).

drug courts. Using a national survey, Matusow et al. found widespread prohibition of buprenorphine and methadone, with neither option allowed in approximately half of drug courts.[262] Furthermore, only one-third of courts allowed participants to start buprenorphine or methadone, as opposed to continuing medication previously prescribed prior to drug court participation. Despite clear evidence by this time that MAT is the most effective treatment for opioid addiction, including evidence that the medications prevent relapse among people with involvement in the criminal justice system, and may therefore prevent re-incarceration, a large portion of drug court participants with opioid addiction were being denied access. An even more recent study found that of criminal justice participants referred for OUD treatment, only 20 percent were referred for treatment with buprenorphine or methadone, the gold standard of care for OUD.[263] And of referrals from the criminal justice system for OUD treatment, referrals from drug courts were significantly less likely than referrals from jails and prisons to include buprenorphine or methadone.[263] Yet, unlike jails and prisons, the purpose of drug courts is to engage people in and monitor treatment.

The reasons found by Matusow et al. for drug court prohibitions of buprenorphine and methadone varied somewhat by medication and court location. For example, rural courts were more likely than urban courts to say that buprenorphine prohibitions were related to lack of providers.[262] Common reasons for denying buprenorphine and methadone treatment included the following: MAT was against drug court policy, probably a catchall for "we just don't like it"; cost; participants had already completely detoxed prior to starting drug court; and risk of diversion.[262] The study also confirmed something I had suspected for some time: widespread misconceptions about agonist medications exist in the criminal justice system. For example, Matusow et al. found almost half of drug court staff were unsure whether buprenorphine prevents relapse, and two-thirds were unsure whether methadone prevents relapse. Over one-quarter believed that methadone "rewards drug users" for drug use. One might not expect criminal justice personnel in general to be up to speed on the latest scientific evidence about addiction treatment, but remember that drug courts are specifically created to assist people with addiction treatment.

In 2016, I decided to study the drug court treatment landscape in Indiana. I believed policy makers and public health scholars needed a deeper understanding of the anti-MAT attitudes and policies in drug courts, including how decisions were made in courts, the role of court treatment teams in providing treatment, and how judges get their information about medications. Then armed with this information, policy makers could start to address some of the treatment gaps in drug courts. Broadly speaking, my results confirmed the results of Matusow et al., albeit six years later and in one Midwestern state. But I discovered some new information that helped me understand how misconceptions about MAT arise, spread, and persist in drug courts.

First, treatment-related decisions are made by teams headed by judges who rarely acknowledge their own powers of persuasion. For example, Judge Jackson said: "If there are eleven people on the team that have to have a vote, then I have eleven votes, I guess. But I'm not one that has extensive knowledge of treatment services and things like that, so all the non–mental health professionals and non–substance abuse treatment professionals are certainly going to rely on the experts for their recommendations." Yet despite such claims of humility, throughout interviews judges clearly revealed the powerful role they held on treatment teams, revealing how their own views impact other team members. For example, after describing her supposed deference to treatment providers, Judge Ruiz said, "[So] nobody's on methadone in drug court. I don't allow that."

When judges disapprove of MAT, it can be very difficult for other treatment team members to sway them. The following quote from Judge Noble exemplifies this difficulty: "Probably up until this year we've had a pretty strong bias against medication-assisted treatment, and that's probably been largely because of my biases . . . [but] as it stands now, I suppose that if the treatment folks are recommending medication-assisted treatment and the participant is open to the treatment, then I'm probably going to go along with it."

Judge Barron revealingly states, "I . . . we, we allow the clients to use [Suboxone] short term to age them from a more serious drug and addiction process and kind of bring them down slowly. But whether it's Suboxone or whether it's methadone, I am not a fan of marginalizing our clients for life and saying that we're going to cast them away as lost souls, and we're just basically going to drug them for life. If you're going to use Suboxone, or you're going to use methadone, [or] you're going to use some type of pharmacological response to addiction, it needs to be short term." Note the frequent use of the word "I" rather than "we." While giving lip service to respecting clinical experts, Judge Barron is making treatment decisions based on personal beliefs, namely that MAT is harmful and prevents true recovery.

Some judges feel they have special knowledge about addiction that community clinicians, especially MAT physicians, lack. After all, drug court judges see their participants weekly in a pseudoparental relationship, learning about the participants' family, friends, employment, and motivations, while physicians see a patient monthly for maybe half an hour in a relationship that is formal and at arm's length. As a result, some judges feel clinicians must first prove themselves as truly knowledgeable addiction specialists before they are given deference regarding MAT. Judge Jefferson revealingly stated, "Now I'm willing, personally, as a judge, to have pretty much an open mind about it. If I can find a provider who will give me good, evidence-based reasons for using a particular drug-assisted or medicine-assisted kind of intervention, I'm willing to consider it." Similarly, Judge Hale explained, "It's very difficult to establish quality working relationships with doctors in a drug court setting, and what I mean by that is that I think I have found challenges in finding doctors who really understand about addiction and recovery."

It seems that any effort to expand access to MAT in drug courts must target the judges who oversee drug courts whether or not they acknowledge their own importance. Once one recognizes the role played by the judge's attitudes and beliefs regarding treatments in drug court, stories from interviewees, such as Candace's, really start to make sense. For example, in another series of interviews, Timothy described the turmoil he experienced when he started Suboxone treatment as a participant in a rural drug court last year. Having not been told that the court prohibited Suboxone, he found a buprenorphine provider. Two weeks later, the Suboxone he was legally prescribed appeared in a routine court urine drug screen and was brought to the attention of the judge.

In front of other participants, the judge demanded to know where Timothy received the Suboxone, and Timothy described his participation in treatment through a community physician. In response, the judge threw Timothy into jail for a month. Then Timothy's mother, whom I also interviewed, did something I rarely hear interviewees doing: she found an attorney to fight the judge. The attorney argued that the denial of Timothy's medication and the jail sanction violated the Americans with Disabilities Act. The judge was not persuaded. Then, like a miracle, the judge was replaced. He had been an interim judge while the court looked for a permanent person for the position. The new judge examined the situation and determined that there was nothing legally wrong with Timothy taking Suboxone. Perhaps she was afraid of a lawsuit targeting the drug court so soon after starting her new position. However, the new judge is still not entirely persuaded of Suboxone's efficacy. Nevertheless, according to Timothy, the judge allows it because it could be helpful, and a legitimate physician is prescribing and overseeing the treatment. To date, Timothy is still in the three-year-long drug court program but unfortunately cannot count the month he spent in jail toward the three years. He takes Suboxone daily as prescribed but believes that the rest of the court treatment team still doesn't view his treatment choice as a proper recovery method. Nevertheless, they defer to the judge's decision.

WHY DO SOME JUDGES harbor extreme antagonism toward MAT? For example, one judge told me Suboxone is no different than heroin or whiskey. Another judge called methadone "a hideous, awful thing." Relatedly, why are other judges neutral toward or even in favor of allowing medication? If judges are to remain key treatment decision-makers, then significantly more research is needed into this topic. But my own study provides some clues.

First of all, some judges are *very*, very worried about abuse or diversion of the medications. The role of such fears in their personal decision-making process was revealed when judges said they might allow Probuphine, a surgical implant that slowly releases buprenorphine in the arm over six months, even when they explicitly banned oral versions of buprenorphine. Unlike oral forms, Probuphine is unlikely to be diverted or abused. Basically, diversion or abuse would require ripping the implant out of one's arm—presumably causing extreme pain—and then somehow getting the buprenorphine out of the implant. When I conducted the study, Sublocade, a once-per-month extended-release injection of buprenorphine provided by a physician, was not yet available, but one could imagine judges feeling more favorably toward this formulation than the oral kind as it is likewise difficult to divert or misuse.

It is not surprising that judges are particularly attuned to something that is itself a criminal activity—medication diversion and misuse. After all, judges have far more training in responding to criminal activity than in providing health care services. It would be unfair of the public to expect otherwise, which is exactly why reforming addiction treatment services in the criminal justice system requires a larger role for medical professionals and a smaller role for judges and other criminal justice personnel in medical decision-making.

At the same time, buprenorphine diversion and misuse is often misunderstood. The very first objection I hear to buprenorphine from judges, probation officers, and law enforcement is that it is sold on the street and has street value, as if that alone makes it an ineffective or dangerous medication. It can be very difficult for criminal justice administrators to understand why something sold on the street can be good for a drug court participant. Relatedly, criminal justice administrators often automatically assume that people purchasing buprenorphine on the street are doing so simply to get high. But when people buy buprenorphine on the street, they are usually not intending to get high. Multiple studies, including my own ongoing study, have identified prevention of withdrawals and limited access to formal treatment as the primary reasons for illicit buprenorphine purchases.[72,232,264–267]

I have asked dozens of interviewees across multiple US states about their experiences with buprenorphine diversion and misuse. Specifically, I ask why people buy buprenorphine on the street. The overwhelming majority says it is to prevent withdrawal symptoms. Rarely do interviewees even identify "trying to get high" as a reason for illicit purchases, let alone as the sole reason for illicit purchases. Of course, some people do purchase buprenorphine to get high, but this fact must be taken with a large grain of salt. Someone regularly using heroin, fentanyl, or prescription painkillers who then takes buprenorphine will feel no euphoria and will become very sick from the combination. He or she will experience precipitated withdrawal symptoms, which as previously noted, are even worse than normal withdrawal symptoms. Therefore, who would buy buprenorphine on the street illicitly to get high? The most likely individual would be opioid naïve, meaning someone who does not regularly take other opioids—in other words, someone whose tolerance is so low that buprenorphine will give them a buzz. But even then, their body will quickly build tolerance, sometimes in just a few days, and they will no longer feel high from the buprenorphine. Furthermore, the street offers much better options for a high, and often at a better price; so overall, buprenorphine would be a strange choice. To use this rationale as the basis of a drug court's policy for banning buprenorphine treatment is misguided and irrational. After all, a drug court participant with severe opioid addiction—exactly the kind of person who would benefit from buprenorphine—is unlikely to be opioid naïve.

Even aside from fears of buprenorphine diversion, some drug court judges fear that monitoring treatment, a key part of their job, would become a logistical challenge if MAT were permitted. One source of this challenge stems from the lack of existing, trusting relationships between drug court treatment teams and local MAT providers. If judges trusted a local provider, then they would leave some of the treatment monitoring in the provider's hands. For example, they would trust the MAT provider to contact the court if the drug court participant was failing to attend treatment. They would trust the MAT provider to prescribe a proper dosage rather than one that is too high or too low. Without this kind of trust, court treatment teams feel that allowing MAT is adding an extra layer of work. In contrast, court treatment teams typically have close relationships with one or two local mental health or addiction treatment clinics, almost always abstinence-based. If this local agency does not provide MAT, and statistically it is unlikely to do so,[20,235] then the judge no longer has a provider whom he or she knows and trusts.

Trust is a particularly important theme in my interviews with judges. Just as there have been unscrupulous physicians prescribing painkillers for the "wrong reasons" or with improper monitoring, so too have there been seedy buprenorphine prescribers and overrun methadone clinics. One judge specifically pointed to a news story describing the arrest of a buprenorphine provider as the basis for the court's policy prohibiting buprenorphine altogether. In contrast, during interviews, judges never revealed distrust of counselors or fears of unscrupulous counselors. In fact, some judges trust counselors so much that they use counselors to vet potential MAT prescribers, to determine physicians' legitimacy and whether they are "philosophically" in line with the court treatment team. Specifically, court teams often look for physicians who express preference for short-term MAT, despite the stronger evidence base for longer-term MAT.[77] This philosophical preference for short-term MAT is reflected in court policies that prohibit drug court participants from graduating while still utilizing MAT. In fact, half of the judges in my study who permitted buprenorphine required participants to stop the treatment quickly, with arbitrary timelines ranging from two weeks to a few months. For example, Judge Pruitt explained that he would permit MAT under the following condition: "[I'll allow it] provided you have the right professional administering it and working to wean them off of it. One of the problems that we saw was that we didn't feel like the people administering them were trying to wean them, or cut back and slowly get them off of this medically assisted treatment, and wanted to keep them on it for, I hate to say it, but basically their financial gain." Any future studies of drug court policies, therefore, must examine not only whether courts permit MAT but also how long courts permit MAT.

On the flip side, not surprisingly, physicians don't necessarily want to work with court teams. As Judge Hawkins noted, "I don't think physicians enjoy having their clients be part of our program. . . . I hate to speak for them, but it puts them in a position where we ask that we're permitted to be able to access all the treatment and monitoring. We require our participants to sign a release, and I'm not sure that the doctors appreciate us snooping around or looking at what's going on. So I . . . we don't have a real good relationship with them, I don't think, throughout the community."

Judges' arbitrary time limitations for using MAT are clear examples of inappropriate medical decision-making by personnel without proper medical credentials. Practicing medicine without a license is illegal in all states, yet judges sometimes appear blind to the fact that they are making medical decisions. For example, Judge Becker stated, "Yeah, it's not a deal where [they can take Suboxone] for ninety days. I mean, I don't pretend to be a doctor, but our theory is, you know, you can't substitute one drug for another. . . . Well, it's up to the doctor, but we want them off as soon as they can get off. . . . I wouldn't say more than the thirty days at most. Typically it's two to three weeks."

Judges' anti-MAT attitudes clearly stem, in part, from disbelief in MAT as an effective treatment, or even as treatment at all. Repeatedly during interviews, judges would call counseling "treatment" but would refer to medication as an adjunct to treatment rather than treatment itself. For example, some judges said that participants could access MAT so long as they were also getting "treatment," meaning counseling. Of course, the terminology "medication-assisted treatment," an antiquated phrasing that suggests medication is either not part of the treatment or is, at best, assisting the "real" treatment (i.e., counseling), doesn't help the situation. Scholars are increasingly choosing to call buprenorphine, methadone, and naltrexone "pharmacotherapy" or "medications for opioid use disorder" instead of MAT, but few people seem to know these terms, limiting their usefulness in conversation.

Importantly, judges also appear to trust support groups as a recovery method more so than MAT, leading nineteen of twenty Indiana drug and veterans' courts in my study to require support group participation for people with opioid addiction. Requiring participants to attend AA, NA, or some other spiritual support group likely violates the First Amendment.[268] Judges readily acknowledged that participants could select their own local support group for this reason. But what if no support groups other than AA or NA exist in the area—a very likely situation in rural counties? Though a few judges permitted online support group attendance, many judges appeared to not have considered this problem, likely resulting in nonspiritual participants being forced, for lack of an alternative, to attend spiritual support groups. Requiring support group participation is also problematic if the local groups stigmatize MAT and the participant is undergoing MAT. As discussed in chapter 2, MAT-related stigma is common in twelve-step groups, and when few local support groups exist, people cannot effectively "shop around" until they find a group with which they are comfortable.

Courts that deny MAT access may eventually find themselves in legal trouble. For one, a blanket prohibition of any medication can be considered prejudging facts before hearing evidence from both sides in a case, especially if no rationale is provided. If the matter is appealed to a higher court, then the higher court may call out the lower court for abusing its power and rendering a baseless decision.[269] Additionally, courts that ban MAT are arguably violating the Americans with Disabilities Act, as already mentioned in Timothy's account. Since some federal courts have interpreted this act to include substance use disorder, preventing effective treatment for a disability could be considered a legal violation.

In fact, in 2019 the Circuit Court of Appeals in the First Circuit found that denying buprenorphine to someone in jail may violate the Americans with Disabilities Act.[270] In that case, a woman who had been successfully undergoing buprenorphine treatment for years was arrested for pocketing cash left at a Walmart register. She was arrested, and the jail refused to continue her buprenorphine treatment. A federal district court heard her case, deciding in her favor, with the higher court later agreeing. In the district court opinion, the judge made the following remarks:

> In a randomized, controlled trial conducted in the Rhode Island correctional system, incarcerated people who were permitted to continue taking their prescribed methadone were seven times more likely to continue treatment after release than were inmates who were forcibly withdrawn from MAT. The evidence of MAT's benefits has become so compelling that it would no longer be possible to conduct the kind of randomized trial that was used in Rhode Island . . . researchers would not

consider it "ethically feasible to deny a group a medication that has such [a] proven track record at improving outcomes."[270]

DRUG COURTS CLEARLY have significant room for improvement. But lest we forget, a large percentage of people in the criminal justice system for drug-related crimes are not in jail, prison, or drug court but rather are on probation. Even though being on probation means you can continue to live at home and attend work, it differs from drug court in some significant ways. Treatment, for one, is not necessarily required, even for addiction-related crimes; however, some judges require it in the terms of probation. When treatment is required, decisions are rarely made by a "treatment team," giving the judge and probation officer a lot of power. For example, until this year in Oregon, probation and parole officers had to approve criminal justice system participants' utilization of methadone or buprenorphine, even when prescribed by a qualified physician.[271,272] Unlike in drug court, relapse while on probation is rarely tolerated, often resulting in immediate incarceration. In contrast, in drug court a series of relapses will lead to termination but not just one or two. Despite even the lack of a veneer of clinical credentials, probation officers make medical decisions—especially when it comes to MAT.

Kristen, who has opioid addiction, was commanded by the judge to attend the local mental health and addiction treatment center as part of her probation terms. That treatment center, chosen because the probation officer was most familiar with it and trusted it, did not offer MAT. Kristen asked the judge if she could attend treatment at a different local center that offered MAT instead. The judge responded, "If your probation officer deems that it is acceptable." To Kristen's knowledge, the probation officer's credentials consisted of a bachelor's degree in criminology, hardly the credentials one needs to assess the validity of different local treatment centers or their treatment modalities. Fortunately, the probation officer did allow Kristen to attend the other treatment center and to start Suboxone. Nevertheless, the probation officer viewed the medication with skepticism, pushing Kristen to quit. Kristen says, "The entire time I was on probation, every time I saw my probation officer, she'd be like, 'Are you going down yet [on the Suboxone dosage]? Are you getting out of there?' Or, 'How close are you to leaving?' She was just very pushy about it and didn't seem to think that it was a good enough program for me. And I've been clean this whole time. It's worked out great for me. I don't see why [she] thinks it's such a bad thing."

Dawn had a similar experience with her probation officer, who technically allowed Suboxone but took regular opportunities to bash the medication and urge Dawn to taper. "My probation officer said it's not clean being on that. She'd [look at me] like I was crazy and disgusting and a drug addict and that was it. And then continue to talk about do I have a plan for when I'm going to get off of [the medication]." When I ask Dawn how such comments made her feel, she says, "You cannot tell me that this isn't helping me, that it's just me trading one drug for another because it's not the same! I got to go to a pharmacy to pick up my prescription and there is nothing scary or unsafe about it. And if my kids are around when I pick it up, they would have no idea [what it is] . . . they would just think I'm picking up my prescription and that it helps Mommy."

Even if people are permitted to access MAT while on probation, the judge or probation officer may not view the treatment center providing MAT as adequate for meeting court-imposed treatment requirements. In such a case, the judge or probation officer sometimes requires the individual to attend two treatment centers at the same time: one that the criminal justice administrator trusts and the other one that the participant actually likes. As mentioned above, trust is an important theme when it comes to criminal justice administrators and MAT providers. The price of distrust is either denial of effective treatment or forcing people in recovery to spend twice as much time and money in treatment centers as necessary. For example, Mark described being required to attend an abstinence-only treatment center with group counseling, individual counseling, and urine drug screens because his probation officer did not trust the quality of counseling and urine drug screens required by the MAT-providing treatment center. The constant driving back and forth is interfering with Mark's construction job—something that he really needs in order to afford the treatments to begin with.

In contrast to their attitudes toward buprenorphine or methadone, criminal justice professionals often exhibit a markedly different attitude toward extended-release naltrexone. In my 2016 study, judges overwhelmingly preferred extended-release naltrexone, sometimes going out of their way during hearings to praise participants doing well on the medication to encourage other court participants to try it. Since extended-release naltrexone cannot be diverted or misused, judges feel more comfortable with it than with the other medications. Nevertheless, four judges in my study still would not let participants graduate on extended-release naltrexone, as if merely utilizing the medication was a sign that you are not fully in recovery. In 2018, my colleagues and I conducted a survey of 135 Indiana court personnel, including judges, that confirmed our suspicion that attitudes toward extended-release naltrexone in that population are better than attitudes toward buprenorphine; and attitudes toward buprenorphine are better than attitudes toward methadone.[273]

Judges' favoritism toward extended-release naltrexone might also be explained by the manufacturer, Alkermes, directly marketing the medication to judges[56] and taking advantage of courts' historical antagonism toward buprenorphine and methadone. In my own study, Judge Janice stated, "We work really closely with the drug rep from Alkermes, which makes the drug, and they've been very supportive in funding us, giving us discounts for some of our people, even providing a month or two or three of free doses to get somebody started where they don't have insurance." But it is exactly that push from judges to get people on extended-release naltrexone that makes some people in recovery hesitant. For example, John, who is treated with buprenorphine, says, "I looked into [Vivitrol] and realized that the makers of Vivitrol were hitting up the court system, kind of like drug reps do at doctors' offices. That made me nervous . . . that kind of freaked me out about it." Given the frequency with which people in recovery negatively experience the criminal justice system, a medication with close ties to judges can unsurprisingly raise a red flag.

THE PATH FORWARD to changing anti-MAT practices in the criminal justice system, including in drug courts, will not be easy. Drug courts often operate as isolated islands, with treatment teams rarely including physicians and judges ruling with no medical experience. Locals rarely know how drug courts operate or even what they are. Many Americans don't care about access to effective medical treatment in prisons and jails when so many law-abiding citizens outside of the penal system cannot access or pay for their own health care as it is. But changes in the criminal justice system, a uniquely isolated health care sector, require public awareness.

When drug court judges wear multiple hats (e.g., as both the felony court judge and the drug court judge), the public may fail to properly evaluate judges' roles with respect to the drug court. Therefore, states providing funding to drug courts should require them to publicly post treatment-related policies, the names and roles of court treatment team members, program graduation rates, and other basic data annually on publicly available websites. The public, including local health care practitioners, cannot possibly comment on court policies or effectively volunteer their services to the court without such information. Policy makers and researchers can then use such public data to compare policies and outcomes across jurisdictions.

Voluntary professional organizations, such as the National Association of Drug Court Professionals (NADCP), should also more strongly encourage judges to permit MAT and dissuade them from making treatment-related decisions. In fact, almost every judge whom I interviewed stated that he or she attends the NADCP national conference annually, describing the conference very positively. In many cases, it is the primary addiction-related education received by judges. Given the pedestal on which many judges seem to hold the NADCP, state and federal governments should partner with the organization when instituting reforms in drug courts.

Money, of course, is also a potential policy lever. Drug courts, prisons, and jails all get funding from some government source, whether local, state, or federal, and that funding can have strings attached. In fact, the federal government under the Obama administration instituted a new policy wherein drug courts that prohibit MAT access would be stripped of federal funding.[274] But my study found that few Indiana drug courts rely on federal funding, making state or local funding a potentially more effective policy lever. Judges also overwhelmingly disagreed with the idea of tying funding to local court policies, viewing the federal government as encroaching on their authority. Nevertheless, tying funding to MAT signals the importance of MAT as a recovery method. For example, Judge Marion explained, "We're all a little skeptical of [MAT] around here. But I know from going to the NADCP meetings, and not that we get any federal funding, but federal funding is tied to it . . . the federal government will not fund anything if we don't allow medically assisted treatment. . . . It means that, well, there's somebody that thinks that it's pretty important."

Finally, policy makers should critically reexamine the purpose of drug courts. Clearly, drug court participation is preferable to incarceration, but that does not mean that our current approach to drug courts is best. Perhaps after more than three decades the current drug court model should be flipped on its head with drug courts restricted to serving two purposes: monitoring treatment compliance and connecting participants to wraparound services.

In fact, a court "treatment" team, at least as currently conceptualized, wouldn't really be needed at all. Instead, all medical decisions, including the type and frequency of treatment, would be made by counselors and physicians outside of the court who would then inform the court staff about progress in treatment. The judge would enforce sanctions in the event of lack of treatment participation, but only after the court case manager addresses potential barriers to treatment access, such as insurance or transportation.

In this hypothetical model, courts would not even conduct urine drug screens because a positive drug screen may simply signal that the current treatment plan needs adjustment—a decision better left in the hands of medical professionals. Relatedly, judges would only sanction participants for failure to attend treatment rather than for relapse, which would be understood as a symptom of the medical condition. The court case manager would connect participants to wraparound services, such as employment or housing.

So far I have interviewed only a few courageous drug court judges taking this approach. But many seem open to the idea, so long as they can be convinced that local MAT providers are trustworthy. Perhaps a state agency should create a preapproved list of clinicians for treating drug court participants, essentially granting a seal of approval on which judges and court staff could base their ever-important trust. Preapproval could include such factors as having had no disciplinary action from a state licensing board, allowing or providing all forms of MAT, and/or quality indicators, so long as the quality indicators are based on solid research. By having a preapproved list of providers, rather than just one or two agencies with whom the drug court collaborates, participants would also have greater choice in treatment, an important benefit since liking your treatment provider (a component of "therapeutic alliance") is a strong predictor of continuing treatment.[275]

Finally, even if problem-solving courts operate on an ideal model wherein their role is limited to monitoring and enforcement, health care costs may still serve as a barrier to participants accessing MAT. For example, despite her openness to MAT, one Florida judge explained to me that hardly anyone in her court utilizes MAT because local MAT providers do not accept Medicaid and many individuals in her court program are ineligible for Medicaid. The latter point confused me. Do drug court participants have a high income in her jurisdiction? Then she explained that under Governor Rick Scott, Florida refused to expand Medicaid coverage, preventing single young men from accessing Medicaid despite being poor. She described one participant who had lost custody of his child due to drug use but was motivated to participate in treatment as a path to regaining custody. Unfortunately, by losing custody of his child, he also lost his eligibility for Medicaid in Florida, because he was no longer legally a parent. In contrast, in states that expanded Medicaid, anyone below 133 percent of the federal poverty limit can access Medicaid, regardless of their gender or parental status.[276]

In Florida, some providers can access other sources of public funds. One source of funding repeatedly mentioned in interviews is a special grant available for Vivitrol but no other forms of MAT. However, one judge with whom I spoke believes it's unconscionable to send drug court participants to Vivitrol providers in a climate of uncertain funding. What happens when the funding runs out, the participant's cravings reappear, and the participant, who is no longer tolerant, overdoses?

In 2019, I began collaborating with Florida's Office of the State Courts Administrator, which has a new awareness campaign educating judges and court staff about the benefits of MAT and person-centered care. So far, I am encouraged by what I have seen, such as judges in some jurisdictions consciously increasing deference to provider decisions, but a long road still lies ahead, especially in states without an agency championing evidence-based practices in courts.

7

LEARNING FROM OTHER COUNTRIES

GIVEN OUR RELATIVELY isolated geographic location, bordered by an ocean on each side and only two other countries, one above and another below, Americans sometimes forget to examine how other nations deal with complex problems. I remember as a law student being struck by how no time in mandatory law classes was spent examining the laws of other nations, except the laws of England when they directly influenced our own history. Such an introspective view of any social science subject, including health care services, is a weakness rather than a strength, especially when trying to solve complex problems resistant to simple solutions. After all, we are not the only country that has faced opioid-related health crises. Many European countries and Asian countries have had similar dilemmas, including HIV outbreaks from injection drug use. Their experiences can help us critically examine American approaches to the opioid overdose crisis.

Selecting a handful of countries to compare out of all possible nations in the world is a daunting task. Some arbitrary decision-making would undoubtedly influence any scholar. After all, methadone is available as addiction treatment in at least forty-eight countries and buprenorphine in at least thirty-four countries.[277] With that disclaimer in mind, I selected the following countries' health services, laws, and policies with respect to addiction treatment and medication-assisted treatment: France, the United Kingdom (UK), Portugal, and Russia. Russia is the foil in the plot—an example of a country whose policies toward opioid addiction are even less evidence-based than our own, resulting in unnecessary human suffering. On the other hand, France, the UK, and Portugal each have either innovative or evidence-based approaches as dominant features of their addiction treatment policies. Their status in the Organisation for Economic Co-operation and Development, a club of wealthy, stable nations, makes them comparable in many ways to our own. Furthermore, their treatment services are widely available, providing vast amounts of data for health service researchers to examine. For example, a 2007 cross-national study found that only 7 percent of North Americans with opioid addiction were in treatment, while 59 percent of Europeans with opioid addiction were in treatment.[277]

The UK, France, and Portugal are also part of the European Union (EU), though the UK will soon be leaving it. Although health-related policies are primarily set by individual EU member nations, as a regulatory body the EU strongly influences its nations.[278] Since the 1990s, the EU has generally favored harm reduction and evidence-based approaches to drug problems rather than supply-side approaches,[278] in stark contrast to the United States. The EU's adoption of harm reduction policies was strongly influenced by the visible failure of American-style policies.[279] In fact, the United States has served as a model of *disfavored* approaches, with EU policy makers criticizing our heavy criminalization of minor drug possession offenses ("zero-tolerance policies"), few syringe exchange programs, and nonexistent safe legal injection sites.[278,279] Indicating its appreciation for harm reduction and evidence-based approaches to drug problems, the EU maintains a "best practices portal" run by its European Monitoring Centre for Drugs and Drug Addiction. With user-friendly features, it rates the evidence for different practices, even encouraging heroin-assisted treatment for people who continue to relapse following multiple attempts of MAT,[280] something one could hardly imagine the United States encouraging on government-run websites.

As a multinational regulatory body, the EU has been a drug policy pioneer. Within the EU, Portugal has been particularly innovative.[278] In 2001, it became the first European nation to decriminalize possession and use of all drugs, including heroin. The shift was largely a cost-saving measure, since incarcerating people was demonstrably inefficient and ineffective.[278] It is worth noting that fiscal arguments for even controversial policy changes can cut across many political and cultural barriers, as everyone hates government waste of taxpayer money.

Although often misunderstood, Portugal's law did not legalize drugs like heroin, meaning that if you want heroin, you still must go through the black market to get it. Additionally, penalties for drug trafficking are still stringently enforced. In contrast, penalties for possession and use were eliminated, codifying an already existing practice of minimal enforcement for possession and use. Rather than dramatically shifting Portugal's existing policies, the 2001 law built upon the sentiments found in previous laws with a health-oriented approach.[281] For example, an earlier law from 1993 stated, "The drug consumer is sanctioned by current law in a quasi-symbolic manner, in which the contact with the formal justice system is designed to encourage him or her to seek treatment."[282] The law further stated that occasional drug users "should, above all, not be labeled or marginalized" and allowed for flexibility in dismissing charges against occasional users.[282] From 1993 to 2001, almost no one arrested for drug possession or use was incarcerated.[281]

Portugal's 2001 law reflected its previous policy sentiments,[281] except now *all* penalties for possession and use were eliminated, with possession defined as an amount of drugs for up to ten days of use.[283] No distinction was made between different types of drugs or private versus public use. The law applied equally to heroin and misuse of legally obtained prescription opioids.

People caught possessing fewer than ten days' worth of illicit drugs must appear before a district-level Commission for the Dissuasion of Drug Addiction, wherein police refer people to treatment. If the individual is found to be not addicted or does not agree to treatment, then the commission may, at its discretion, impose a monetary or nonmonetary sanction, such as mandatory reporting to the commission, but the nonmonetary sanction cannot include prison. The commission also cannot mandate compulsory treatment. Importantly, the commission has great flexibility in determining whether to impose a sanction, including the type of sanction, and may consider an individual's health, financial status, and other factors. Portugal's law, then, is almost 180 degrees opposite to American mandatory minimum sentencing laws, which require judges to implement severe penalties for drug possession with limited flexibility in decision-making.

Incarceration in the United States as a penalty is the norm for drug-related crimes, with diversion to treatment being the exception, such as when a drug court exists in the county. In contrast, in Portugal, diversion to treatment is the norm and the overarching goal of the law. Furthermore, the Portuguese system of diversion pushes the individual out of the criminal justice system, whereas in American drug courts, the individual is still firmly entrenched in the criminal justice system. Nevertheless, Portugal's decriminalization law is still imperfect; many people caught under the law are not actually addicted or in need of treatment but rather occasional cannabis users.[281] Having such people processed before the commission arguably wastes resources that could be better devoted to people who really need help.

Sophisticated analyses* of the impacts of drug decriminalization on drug use rates in Portugal have found no significant change

* Analyzing pre- and postdecriminalization effects in Portugal is especially complicated for the following reasons: trafficking penalties did not change but possession/use penalties disappeared; the decriminalization law was actually a relatively minor change to existing practices; and cannabis experimentation was already increasing prior to decriminalization.

in drug use between pre- and postdecriminalization, except perhaps in short-term cannabis experimentation.[281] Importantly, heavy drug use has not increased.[281] American politicians and political organizations routinely fear that decriminalization will lead to increased drug use, but this is based on the theory that the level of punishment for an illegal action directly relates to the likelihood of engaging in the action, known as the theory of deterrence. Over time, this theory has been contested by empirical evidence that the likelihood of being caught is far more important at preventing criminal activity than the severity of the punishment,[284] a fact the US government explicitly acknowledges through National Institute of Justice publications.[285] And deterrence theory is likely more applicable to experimentation or occasional drug use than compulsive, regular drug use. As discussed earlier, punishment is largely ineffective for drug addiction, which by definition is the compulsive use of substances *despite* negative consequences.

With respect to addiction treatment, Portugal's decriminalization law is associated with a more than 30 percent increase in the number of people in outpatient treatment and an almost 50 percent increase in the number of treatment centers available nationally over a decade.[281] Of people in outpatient treatment, three-quarters are undergoing MAT, specifically buprenorphine or methadone treatment.[281] The treatment increase is both welcome and expected since the primary purpose of the decriminalization law was to decrease stigma and shift people out of incarceration into evidence-based treatment. Relatedly, new HIV cases among injection drug users dropped precipitously (by about 90 percent) in Portugal over the same time period, though new HIV cases also dropped across the EU as a whole.[281]

METHADONE AND BUPRENORPHINE treatment services in France and England also look dramatically different from those in the United States, largely due to regulations that have allowed MAT to become part of mainstream medicine. Even though they remain somewhat controversial treatments, health care providers and policy makers in France and England appear to have a better understanding of agonist treatment risks and benefits than their counterparts here.

In France, methadone treatment begins at a specialized addiction treatment center; but unlike in the United States, as soon as the individual is stabilized, he or she is transferred to a general practitioner to continue treatment.[286] Once transferred, the patient typically picks up his or her methadone biweekly at a community pharmacy rather than daily, preventing unnecessary travel time and interference with work or family obligations.[286]

Buprenorphine treatment is even easier to access in France than methadone treatment. It is the opioid addiction treatment for which France is best known. The first buprenorphine prescription can be initiated by a French general practitioner and then picked up monthly at the community pharmacy,[286] which largely resembles buprenorphine treatment practices in the United States. But unlike the US health care provider, the French general practitioner faces no patient limits or special education requirements, although many physicians voluntarily seek out special education.[64] Nevertheless, some scholars argue that increased training availability is important for French physicians[287] because some physicians may inappropriately prescribe buprenorphine doses that are too low or lack awareness of national prescribing guidelines.[288]

In the early 1990s, France was facing its own opioid crisis. Injection drug use, especially heroin, accounted for up to 35 percent of new HIV cases.[289] Largely in response to this crisis, France became the first EU nation to approve buprenorphine treatment for opioid addiction, hoping it would decrease HIV rates and overdose deaths.[64] Prior to buprenorphine's approval, French general practitioners had limited involvement in addiction treatment, typically preferring to refer patients to specialists instead. Like in the United States, addiction treatment specialists, namely psychiatrists, were not widely available, thereby limiting the number of patients who could access specialist services. With HIV spreading, such reliance on specialists appeared impractical.

After approving buprenorphine for addiction treatment, France strongly encouraged general practitioners to treat patients with opioid addiction, and buprenorphine made it possible to do so without first referring patients out to a specialist. The French government encouraged general practitioners to prescribe buprenorphine in part because they realized that general practitioners were already health service providers for HIV/AIDS,[289] the most pressing health crisis at the time. As a result, between 1995 and 2003, the number of people in agonist treatment, meaning treatment with buprenorphine or methadone, increased by 95 percent, with buprenorphine representing 80 percent of all agonist treatments.[64] Over 90 percent of buprenorphine was prescribed by general practitioners, in stark contrast to the United States, where only 3 percent of primary care physicians even hold a DATA waiver.[93] It appears that general practitioners (or primary care physicians) can have a profound impact on opioid addiction treatment access. By 2007, 20 percent of all French physicians were prescribing buprenorphine to treat opioid addiction,[64] almost seven times the percentage of US physicians in 2015 who held a DATA waiver—many of whom do not even prescribe buprenorphine despite the ability to do so.[93]

A number of legal, financial, and cultural explanations exist for why buprenorphine treatment is so popular in France, including among general practitioners. As mentioned above, the ability to initiate the prescription without referring out first is certainly a large factor, as is the lack of special certifications, waivers, education, or patient limits. Insurance reimbursement also plays an important role in promoting buprenorphine treatment, in stark contrast to the United States where it is commonly cited as a prescribing barrier.[178]

More than 90 percent of French people have social insurance, which is especially important for the poor or marginalized. General practitioners receive 100 percent reimbursement for management of chronic diseases from the social insurance, as opposed to 65 percent for other ordinary consultations, meaning that treatment for opioid addiction, a chronic condition, is fully reimbursed.[64] Therefore, French physicians are more incentivized to treat opioid addiction than many other serious health conditions. And the treatment is long-term, with more than 80 percent of patients continuing buprenorphine for at least two years.[64,290] Additionally, a dense network of psychosocial support exists, fully covered by the social insurance, to which general practitioners can refer patients.[64] Of course, if they need to, general practitioners can still refer complex patients out to specialists whose costs are fully covered by social insurance. For decades, the French government has formally helped organize such cooperation between general practitioners and specialists through injection drug use and HIV treatment networks.

How has increased buprenorphine treatment availability affected French people with opioid addiction? Multiple studies have demonstrated significant decreases in social vulnerability measures, including unemployment and homelessness, directly related to the buprenorphine treatment. Most importantly, within a few years of buprenorphine's approval, opioid overdose deaths decreased by about 80 percent.[64,290] Heroin and benzodiazepine utilization likewise decreased by about 50 percent among French people in buprenorphine treatment.[290]

With such widespread buprenorphine prescribing in France, one might fear widespread diversion. In fact, an estimated 10 to 20 percent of patients in France being treated with buprenorphine participate in buprenorphine misuse, diversion, pharmacy shopping, or doctor shopping at some point during treatment.[64,290] However, when buprenorphine is prescribed at doses higher than 8 mg, doctor and pharmacy shopping appear rare, suggesting that at least some illicit access is driven by suboptimal dosages.[64] Furthermore, deaths from buprenorphine overdose are very rare, and any buprenorphine-related deaths involved on average three other psychotropic medications, typically benzodiazepines, causing researchers to conclude that the causal role of buprenorphine in these deaths is questionable.[64] Likewise, reported adverse reactions from buprenorphine treatment in France are rare.[290] After reviewing dozens of studies on the role of buprenorphine access in France's overdose rate, as well as diversion rates, one researcher concludes, "From a public health perspective, it is difficult to imagine doing any better when comparing with other regions in Europe, North America, and Australia."[64] He further argues that ideally diversion, doctor-shopping, and pharmacy-shopping rates should decrease, but it is important not to create "unexpected adverse consequences from measures intended to do better."[64] Basically, he argues against limiting buprenorphine availability in an attempt to decrease diversion.

One of the key differences in treatment between France and the United States is the role of the community pharmacy and pharmacist. In the United States, multiple interviewees have described difficulty finding a pharmacy that carries buprenorphine. When picking up the medication, interviewees sometimes describe feeling stigmatized, as if they suddenly receive the label of "drug addict" upon mentioning the prescription name. Furthermore, to my knowledge buprenorphine prescribers in the United States typically have little or no direct communication with the pharmacist dispensing the medication. Yet in France the community pharmacist has been well integrated within the treatment team, collaborating with buprenorphine-prescribing and methadone-prescribing physicians.

Just a few years after buprenorphine was legalized in France, a study in one region found that 80 percent of pharmacists agreed to dispense buprenorphine.[291] A more recent study from 2013 found that 95 percent of pharmacies in the Lille region of France dispensed buprenorphine and methadone, with approximately 80 percent of surveyed pharmacists believing agonist treatment benefited the individual and/or society.[286] In 2005, a study found that over half of general practitioners actively collaborated with pharmacists in managing patients undergoing buprenorphine treatment.[292] Pharmacists in France are reported to engage in the following activities: educating patients about opioid addiction, agonist treatment benefits and risks, proper use of the medication, safe storage away from children, and potential drug interactions; contacting the general practitioner if patients report cravings or withdrawal symptoms; screening for misuse and potential diversion; and, of course, dispensing the medication.[286] Approximately half of the pharmacies in the 2013 study had an isolated area for private consultation between the pharmacist and patient, something the authors would like to see in every pharmacy.[286]

It seems that in the United States we have underestimated the role that community pharmacists can play in addiction treatment. While some pharmacists undoubtedly stigmatize people with opioid addiction, there are likely many pharmacists in the United States who would be willing to step up to the plate but have not been offered the opportunity to do so. For example, one session packed with pharmacists at a recent addiction conference I attended explored how they could play a larger role in addressing the opioid overdose epidemic, with ideas ranging from dispensing MAT to providing free syringes and naloxone.

HEROIN HAS HAD a strong presence in Russia ever since smuggling routes were established to and from Afghanistan after the fall of the Soviet Union.[293,294] Today it is the largest heroin market in Europe.[295] Increasing heroin injection rates have caused Russia to have one of the highest HIV infection rates in the world, with 70–80 percent[295] of new cases related to injection drug use (seven times the world average).[293] Unfortunately, much of the tragedy is preventable. Agonist treatment and syringe exchange programs are well known to limit the spread of HIV, with methadone access decreasing HIV infection rates by as much as 54 percent;[296] but buprenorphine and methadone treatment are illegal in Russia, while syringe exchange programs are very limited.[293] High incarceration rates of drug users in Russia further contribute to the spread of HIV by concentrating people who inject drugs and have HIV in one area.[294]

Russia serves as an example of prioritizing abstinence-only ideology to the detriment of drug users and the general population. One study argues that if attitudes in Russia toward agonist treatment were to change, agonist treatment could be implemented fairly quickly given existing health infrastructure.[293] Access to health care is a constitutional right and Russians obtain mandatory health insurance paid for through taxation and payroll contributions.[293] A multilevel health service system already exists with specialized "narcology" hospitals wherein addiction is treated.[293] Narcologists, the name for psychiatrists in Russia who treat addiction, provide the bulk of the treatment in these hospitals. Unfortunately, current narcology hospital treatment for opioid addiction is largely ineffective, consisting of detoxification and counseling followed by oral naltrexone treatment, with minimal follow-up or connection to community resources.[293] Interestingly, Russia is one of the few nations in the world, other than the United States, where policy makers and health practitioners often take a particularly rosy view toward naltrexone, which is rarely utilized for opioid addiction in most other nations.[277] This perspective is likely influenced by historic attitudes disfavoring agonist treatments and favoring abstinence-only treatment in both nations.

Patients in Russian narcology hospitals report an overwhelming health service focus on treating withdrawal symptoms with limited management of cravings.[295] Such results are unsurprising, given that agonist treatment is particularly effective at managing cravings yet unavailable. Nevertheless, many health providers in Russia do not see a problem. A study of Russian narcologists found widespread negative attitudes toward agonist treatments (i.e., buprenorphine and methadone) and a consensus that treatment as currently provided was sufficient.[297] The primary textbook used by narcologists calls methadone "misguided,"[297] with no scientific evidence provided for this assertion; instead, the textbook relies on the prestigious, hierarchical position of the author. Such negative attitudes toward agonist treatments are reinforced by government memoranda that attack methadone treatment and are then circulated among narcology hospital employees.[297]

One such memorandum, signed by a former head of the Russian Society of Psychiatrists, asks employees to "say no to methadone." It goes on to explain, "The effective way to solve the problem of drug addiction treatment is an intensive search for and introduction of new methods and means that focus on complete cessation of drug use by patients with addiction, their socialization into a new lifestyle free from drugs, but not on exchanging from one drug to another."[297] Furthermore, the authors construct a narrative in which methadone is an attack on traditional Russian moral values by the enemy, in other words, the West. Some physicians claim to represent the medical view of the Russian Orthodox church, arguing that allowing methadone for treatment purposes is the first step toward immoral legalization of drugs.[297] The few narcologists who publicly support agonist treatment are sometimes targeted by government prosecutors for their beliefs.[297] Unfortunately, few opportunities exist for most Russian narcologists to change their views, since opposing perspectives are repressed, domestic educational opportunities about agonist treatments are limited, and educational travel to foreign countries is minimal.[297]

Nevertheless, adding agonist treatment to the tool kit already in use at narcology hospitals, plus into community-based treatment centers, is feasible. Until recently, Ukraine, which had a similar health care infrastructure to that of Russia, permitted agonist treatment with successful results,[298] even though agonist treatment utilization there remained low due to stigma.[299] Unfortunately, Russia's recent control of Crimea has likely been deadly for some Ukrainians recovering from opioid addiction. Following the Crimean invasion, Russia announced plans to cease buprenorphine and methadone treatment in the regions it occupied.[300] In response, one Ukrainian quoted in *The Lancet* said, "Without substitution therapy, I will die. And that is not me just being dramatic or using a figure of speech, I will literally die. So will many others."[300] Russia's negative attitudes toward agonist treatment also influence some other former Soviet nations, such as Uzbekistan and Turkmenistan, which likewise ban agonist treatment for opioid addiction.[294]

Further exemplifying Russia's distrust of harm reduction practices, the nation has no diversion programs for people convicted of drug-related crimes, including no drug courts.[301] Minor drug crimes, including possession of tiny amounts of drugs, such as residue in a syringe, result in lengthy incarceration terms.[300] As easy as it is to criticize Russia's approach toward drug users, let us not forget that Russia's policies have much in common with historic US policies, which likewise emphasized a criminal justice rather than a public health approach to drug problems.[297]

WHEREAS AGONIST TREATMENT is illegal in Russia, the UK government recognizes methadone and buprenorphine as the most important population-level interventions to help people recover from opioid addiction.[302] These medications are considered part of a comprehensive tool kit, along with psychosocial services and peer supports. The focus on agonist treatment has resulted in three quarters of people in UK addiction treatment services undergoing methadone or buprenorphine treatment, with methadone treatment as the preeminent approach.[302] Nevertheless, some health care providers, policy makers, and advocates in the UK are concerned with long-term use of agonists, hoping that people will eventually experience medication-free recovery.[302]

Like in France, general practitioners are the "heart" of treatment services for opioid addiction in the UK.[303] Uniquely, the UK government persuades general practitioners to initiate patients on methadone treatment. In contrast, methadone in France must first be prescribed in specialized treatment centers; in the United States it can only be prescribed in methadone clinics.[303] In the UK, methadone treatment is dispensed daily, weekly, biweekly, or monthly by community pharmacists, depending on the prescription written by the general practitioner. Therefore, the results of methadone prescribing by general practitioners in the UK are particularly interesting to health service researchers, including myself. After all, in the United States the risks of prescribing methadone to people with opioid addiction have been considered too high for general practitioners who have insufficient education, staffing, or other supportive resources.

One might expect that general practitioners in the UK would avoid voluntarily treating patients with methadone despite the ability to do so. After all, these are traditionally "difficult" patients, often with co-occurring mental health disorders, polydrug use, and vulnerable living situations, such as homelessness. Yet a 2005 national study of UK general practitioners found that half had treated a patient with opioid addiction over a one-month period.[303] Of those practitioners who did not actively treat opioid addiction, the primary reasons were lack of patient need, lack of patient interest, or patients already seeing a different practitioner, rather than lack of physician interest.[303]

In the UK, general practitioners do not have restrictions on the number of patients to whom they can prescribe buprenorphine or methadone. Of course, physicians could implement such restrictions themselves as an office-based policy, but three-quarters of general practitioners surveyed did not limit the number of opioid addiction patients whom they treat with MAT. Interestingly, more than half had formal practice arrangements with specialists, despite the lack of any government regulation requiring such arrangements. Clearly, general practitioners realize when they are out of their depth, and at those times they refer patients to specialists. Of those general practitioners who treated a patient with opioid addiction in the one-month period studied, half had prescribed either methadone or buprenorphine, with methadone dominating, representing 87 percent of prescriptions.[303] About half of the prescriptions were for daily dispensation; the other half were for weekly, biweekly, or monthly dispensation, suggesting that general practitioners can manage a wide range of opioid addiction severity.[303]

It is difficult to overstate how different methadone prescribing looks in the UK relative to the United States. The UK's methadone treatment initiation and management by general practitioners, combined with the frequency with which people are given take-home doses (a decision made by the physician without government intrusion) strongly suggests that UK policy makers trust general practitioners' decision-making expertise. These less stringent methadone prescribing policies also suggest a national preference for harm reduction and low-barrier treatment. Yes, take-home doses make diversion easier; but take-home doses may also improve treatment retention and compliance.[304] The UK's focus then is clearly on improving health service adherence rather than on preventing methadone-related criminal activity.

Why do so many general practitioners in the UK treat opioid addiction? Setting aside the less stringent regulations for prescribing methadone and buprenorphine, which clearly have a strong influence, there are other persuasive factors present in the health care system. For example, in some areas, general practitioners who treat opioid addiction receive extra reimbursement for methadone prescribing.[303] In other words, like the French government, the UK government has utilized financial incentives as a useful tool for encouraging opioid addiction treatment. Such incentives may be particularly important for general care practitioners to counteract potential stigma that exists toward opioid addiction patients and to compensate for the extra staff and time utilized in treating this chronic condition. Interestingly, many of the general practitioners who prescribe MAT refer to themselves as "specialist general practitioners," indicating that they have come to view opioid addiction treatment as part of the core health services they provide.[303] Additionally, they work collaboratively with many health care providers, ranging from addiction specialists to psychologists and pharmacists, even if they are not all located in the same building.

Like in France, UK pharmacists play an important role in opioid addiction treatment too, not only by dispensing medication but also by educating patients and serving as liaisons between providers and patients when necessary. For example, community pharmacies are legal dispensers of syringes to active drug users. If a pharmacist notices that a patient picking up methadone is also picking up syringes, indicating ongoing opioid misuse, then the pharmacist is encouraged to ask the patient's permission to speak with the general practitioner about escalation of treatment services.[305]

Attitudes of pharmacists in England are generally favorable toward agonist treatments and have become more so over time.[306] As is common in studies of stigma among health care practitioners, it appears that once pharmacists spend more time with people recovering from opioid addiction, they tend to reexamine long-held stigmatizing beliefs and adopt more positive ones. Similarly, increased contact between physicians and drug users in France has caused a decrease in stigmatizing attitudes toward people with opioid addiction among French physicians.[289]

In 2017, the UK Department of Health published clinical guidelines for opioid addiction treatment. Though these guidelines do not themselves have the force of law, other laws require clinicians to be familiar with and to try to implement the guidelines.[305] Therefore, they are persuasive documents for providers of health services for opioid addiction. The guidelines tell practitioners to work collaboratively with the patient to identify recovery goals that are far broader than abstinence from drug use, including improving family relationships and social networks. "Attaining controlled drug, non-dependent, or non-problematic drug use" is even stated as a legitimate goal if the patient does not want abstinence.[305] Interestingly, the guidelines explicitly state that MAT prescribers and psychosocial providers should be on the same page regarding the patients' goals. Relatedly, access to MAT should not be contingent on psychosocial services, with each tool only utilized if the patient feels it is appropriate to his or her needs. Fortunately, the US Department of Health and Human Services agrees with this recommendation too, not that I see it followed in practice much.[23]

The guidelines recommend naltrexone for patients who have a strong motivation for abstinence-only treatment or who want ongoing support following withdrawal from other forms of MAT. Naltrexone is not viewed as a "better" alternate to opioid-containing buprenorphine or methadone; it is just another option that a patient can choose. Two sentences jump out at me—sentences that I would like posted on every US addiction treatment provider's desk:

> It is inappropriate, in providing ethical, evidence-based treatment, for services to create a sense that those opting for [methadone or buprenorphine] maintenance are making a poorer choice than those opting for an abstinence-oriented or abstinence-based treatment. Equally, prescribing services should not discourage a patient who wishes to pursue detoxification, but should provide the best information on benefits and risks, and support the patient's considered decision.[305]

As indicated above, the guidelines encourage person-centered care in a variety of ways. For example, if patients do not wish to abstain from drugs, then practitioners should provide them with knowledge about harm reduction, indicating strong consideration for patient preferences and values. For patients in rural areas or with difficulty accessing public transportation, practitioners are told to provide flexible appointment spots and to avoid peremptory discharge for missed appointments. It should be noted that these person-centered recommendations are feasible because they are supported by the regulations, especially those that allow for flexible prescribing and take-home schedules, encourage prescribing by general practitioners (who are more likely to be in rural areas than specialists), and permit pharmacy-based syringe and naloxone provision. The UK's clinical guidelines are an important reminder that health care providers work in a complex ecological model of health services, wherein policies matter as much as institutional factors or interpersonal factors in achieving health care goals.[31]

The UK guidelines are replete with descriptions of the importance of therapeutic alliance—the collaborative relationship between the health care provider and the patient.[305] Providing person-centered care is described as a method to achieve therapeutic alliance, which itself is considered a strong predictor of health service retention and compliance,[305] and addiction treatment retention and compliance are strong predictors of health outcomes.[175] Clearly, the UK guidelines' person-centered care approach is compassionate, nonjudgmental, and empathetic, but it is also a very practical approach to achieving improved health outcomes nationally. Historically, US politicians who encouraged addiction treatment over punitive measures were viewed as "soft" or "weak"; however, from an empirical standpoint, respectful, person-centered addiction treatment is a key element of effective health policy.

A discussion of UK addiction treatment policies would be incomplete without an examination of guidelines for treatment within the criminal justice system. Unlike in the United States, where prisons and jails rarely provide MAT access[258] and essentially force incarcerated people to undergo painful detoxification against their will, the UK takes a markedly different stance. The UK encourages MAT continuation and provision in prisons and jails, with seamless connection to follow-up MAT in the community after release.[305] According to national guidelines, detoxification should be available as an option in jails and prisons but only used if desired by the incarcerated individual after careful consideration of the risks and benefits.[305] Furthermore, naloxone should be provided to prisoners upon release.[305] After dozens of interviews with American criminal justice employees and individuals in recovery, I almost laugh when I consider how contrary such a suggestion is to the normal prison and jail practices in the United States.

SEEN SIDE BY SIDE, the French and UK policies and addiction treatment services suggest that general practitioners can and should be actively involved in both methadone and buprenorphine provision, and they should be integrated with specialists in the care of complex patients. The French and UK experiences also suggest that community pharmacists should be part of the core health care team. As mentioned previously, the UK's general practitioners overwhelmingly prescribe methadone while France's general practitioners overwhelmingly prescribe buprenorphine. In both cases, there is little doubt that general practitioners are capable of caring for a large swath of the population. The Portuguese experience teaches that decriminalization of drug possession and use pushes people into treatment, and when treatment is readily available, overdose and HIV rates decrease. In contrast, studies of Russia exemplify the problems that occur when a morality-based, abstinence-only philosophy dominates addiction treatment policy and services, including HIV care.

In the United States, we are making some progress toward encouraging primary care physicians to treat opioid addiction, but far more progress is needed. Policy changes are a first step. Fortunately, in the last two years federal regulations have allowed physician assistants and nurse practitioners for the first time to prescribe buprenorphine in office-based settings, though sometimes state regulations seriously impede their ability to do so.[207] Nurse practitioners and physician assistants can help lessen the load on primary care physicians, particularly if the two types of professionals work together. Other positive changes have included the ability of a subset of "qualified" physicians to expand their buprenorphine patient limits to 275.

Despite these changes, there have been hardly any improvements in methadone-related policies that currently seriously impede access to care. Patients must still travel long distances, usually daily, to the few methadone clinics that exist in each state. Attitudes toward MAT are slowly becoming more positive, as exemplified by a recent increase in DATA-waivered physicians, but the number of US prescribers has hardly reached the levels of buprenorphine prescribers seen in France. One need only remember a 2017 comment by Tom Price, the former US Secretary of the Department of Health and Human Services under President Trump. Representing the view of many American addiction treatment practitioners, Price called methadone and buprenorphine "just another drug," and then he argued that naltrexone is the only acceptable opioid addiction treatment medication.[307]

SOME PEOPLE WILL repeatedly relapse despite trying methadone or buprenorphine treatment. In the scholarly literature, they are called "refractory" patients. For those people, heroin-assisted treatment and supervised injection sites may be appropriate. The two policies are slightly different, though both aim to reduce potential harm to drug users. Heroin-assisted treatment involves health care providers prescribing heroin to patients, after which patients consume or inject it in a supervised environment, such as the physician's office, or an unsupervised environment, depending on applicable law. Supervised injection sites are typically spaces where people who have obtained heroin on their own, usually meaning illicitly, go to inject. The space offers clean syringes and drug testing kits, as well as a nurse present in the event of an overdose. Often the nurse provides referrals to primary health care and HIV/AIDS or hepatitis C treatment.

Though heroin-assisted treatment and supervised injection sites are illegal in the United States, the evidence base for both has been growing over the last decade in other nations, especially in European countries and Canada.[308] Randomized controlled studies of the two methods have been conducted in a wide range of settings, including Switzerland, Spain, the Netherlands, the UK, and Canada.[309] For refractory patients, both approaches reduce street heroin use and physical and mental health problems.[309] Contrary to public fears, the policies also have a strong significant effect on *reducing* local criminal activity.[309] Importantly, there is no evidence that heroin-assisted treatment or supervised injection sites lead to an increase in injection rates or new drug use.[310]

For almost a century, heroin has been legally prescribed without supervision for refractory patients in the UK, though today few patients receive it.[311] As early as 1920, the UK government permitted physicians to independently decide to prescribe heroin, which would be taken home by the patient and utilized in an undisclosed location.[309] A 1920s UK Ministry of Health report recommended its use for people who cannot safely withdraw from opioids or who "are capable of leading a fairly normal and useful life, so long as they take a certain quantity, usually small, of their drug of addiction, but not otherwise."[309] This advice was issued prior to the existence of methadone or buprenorphine as a treatment. As a result, heroin prescribing was the primary method of opioid addiction treatment in the UK until the 1960s when street heroin use became common, at which point the government began to require physicians who prescribe heroin to have a special license.[309] Most of these licensed physicians were psychiatrists working in specialized addiction clinics.[309] But after studies demonstrated methadone's efficacy in the 1970s, physicians switched from prescribing heroin to prescribing methadone, which had fewer safety risks and a longer half-life.[309]

About twenty years ago, Swiss researchers and policy makers looked to the UK example of heroin-assisted treatment but decided that supervision of heroin injection, rather than take-home dosages, would minimize safety and diversion risks. Therefore, in Switzerland, heroin is both prescribed and injected on-site where its use is observed by a physician or nurse. The supervision and lack of take-home dosages help prevent diversion while keeping the patient safe from overdose. However, heroin is associated with more adverse events than methadone, reinforcing the fact that it is more appropriate as a second-line rather than first-line treatment.[309]

NORTH AMERICA'S FIRST and only government-sanctioned supervised injection site is in Vancouver, Canada. Even though heroin use is illegal in Canada, the safe injection site is viewed favorably by the public and for good reason: it has resulted in a 35 percent drop in local overdose deaths in just two years.[312] The supervised injection site was strategically opened in a location with a large open-air drug market and high HIV rates, as well as high rates of homelessness and low-cost housing. Unlike in Switzerland, the Canadian site's health care providers do not provide heroin or other opioids; rather, they supervise, provide clean syringes, and make referrals for treatment.[313]

Thomas Lawrence, who studies supervised injection sites, argues that it can be very difficult to "import" such controversial policies into new areas, such as the United States.[313] Rather, he suggests that the policy must be "translated" by locals, who adapt it to their needs and culture.[313] Additionally, such policy change occurs after a series of baby steps, such as newspaper articles and local conferences, which may seem unimportant in isolation but are meaningful in combination.[313] In Vancouver, movement toward a government-sanctioned supervised injection site emerged after a local coroner, distraught by the rising opioid overdose deaths, convened a task force that argued for harm reduction measures.[313] The public would not have been responsive to these suggestions but for the growing understanding of addiction as a chronic health condition rather than a moral failing.[313] Ultimately, increased public empathy for the vulnerable population was critical to enacting progressive policies. Not surprisingly, local business owners and the police initially opposed the idea of a supervised injection site, fearing that it would lead to more crime.[313] But health board reports and conferences continued to push the idea, spearheaded by people who had experienced pain associated with addiction, including adult children of drug users.[313] The struggles of drug users were also empathetically explored in local newspaper articles.[313] By 1998, the local public was still deeply divided, with about half supporting a supervised injection site and half opposing it, but attitudes were steadily becoming more progressive even among traditionally conservative politicians.[313]

Although illegal, informal supervised injection sites had existed on and off in the Vancouver area for years, including in a church. But the new government-sanctioned site required the support of local politicians. It was worth the fight, because financial support from the government would be more stable than the shifting, temporary funding from nonprofit organizations upon which informal sites relied. Government support would also lend the site legitimacy, preventing police from targeting the area.[313] Fortunately, the local coroner, mayor, and city drug policy commissioner supported the idea and connected a range of people who cared about health services for drug users.

After much planning, the local health authority applied for the safe injection site through the national health agency, Health Canada, which approved it in 2003.[313] A derelict hotel was demolished and replaced with a $1.2 million government-funded facility, operated by the local health authority with collaboration from other groups, including a housing-focused nonprofit, the police force, and university researchers.[313] Importantly, local police continue to actively support the supervised injection site. In contrast, police in many US jurisdictions target harm reduction program participants with arrest.[310]

In Vancouver, researcher collaboration allowed for robust, ongoing data collection and analysis, which fed back to the public and government. Despite its successes, the safe injection site remains fragile. In recent years, the Canadian federal government attempted to shut down the site, but the Supreme Court of Canada stopped the federal government, arguing that shutting down the supervised injection site would cost lives and increase suffering.[313] Nevertheless, the history of Vancouver's site is informative to US scholars, policy makers, and advocates who would like to see a similar facility opened on this side of the border.

CONCLUSION

IT'S DIFFICULT ENOUGH for a broad range of people interested in and affected by drug policy and health services to agree on the "right" way to reach an end goal. It's even harder when people disagree on the end goals to begin with. After more than 120 in-depth interviews with people in recovery, physicians, counselors, judges, other criminal justice administrators, and policy makers, it is clear to me that these groups often have different pictures of how addiction health services should look. Based on hundreds of hours of interview data and a review of published scholarly studies of addiction health services, I have created a list of the top ten goals I want to see in addiction health services, specifically with respect to opioid addiction treatment and medication-assisted treatment. The United States is already making progress toward some of these goals, in part due to state and federal pressure. Other goals may take decades to achieve.

GOAL 1

Substance use disorder treatment, including MAT, becomes mainstream medicine

If you are reading this book, like me you probably agree that addiction treatment access must increase nationally. But where should people seek treatment? A combination of physicians, counselors, and other providers are needed, working in an integrated team (see chapter 5), but few physicians are currently participating on these teams. Importantly, primary care physicians are left out, or are leaving themselves out, entirely. I have met more than a handful of addiction specialists who argue that primary care physicians are *not* well positioned to treat addiction, but the argument is flawed because it presumes that (1) medical school and residency programs will never change, (2) practicing physicians cannot learn, and (3) primary care physicians cannot collaborate with other behavioral health professionals to fill in knowledge and service gaps.

Obviously, increasing primary care participation in the addiction treatment workforce will not come easily. It will depend on funding, political buy-in, physician interest, destigmatization of addiction, insurance incentives, simplification of privacy laws, and other complex factors. But if primary care physicians are educated and trained to treat addiction with the support of other behavioral health professionals, there are plenty of reasons for them to become the first point of care and even the coordinators of the treatment team. Then when cases are particularly complex, such as when severe co-occurring disorders exist or a patient is pregnant, primary care physicians could send patients to specialists until the patient is stabilized; after which, the patient could return to working with the primary care physician.

Benefits to the patient would include the relatively low stigma associated with seeing a primary care physician relative to other specialists, greater accessibility in most areas to primary care physicians than to specialists, and the holistic view that primary care physicians can provide care by treating co-occurring conditions such as hepatitis C and HIV/AIDS. Specialists, such as psychiatrists, would likewise benefit from this arrangement, which would allow them to focus their time and energy on the most complex patients. Opioid addiction is a relapsing, chronic disease, so the relationship between the primary care physician and specialist would need to be continuous, with the possibility of patients traveling between the providers over time. France and the United Kingdom have already demonstrated the feasibility of this goal.

GOAL 2

Criminal justice administrators stop making health care–related decisions

The criminal justice system is a key provider of health services in the United States (see chapter 6). Ideally, the United States would move toward decriminalization of drug possession and use, much as Portugal has done. Decriminalization would decrease the stigma associated with addiction and push people toward treatment rather than ineffective incarceration. But this is the United States, and I doubt decriminalization would be accepted in many jurisdictions. Therefore, at a minimum we should divert more people convicted of addiction-related crimes into drug courts and similar programs.

There is little doubt that drug courts are more effective at preventing re-incarceration relative to stints in jail or prison. In other words, diversion works; but is it working well enough? I have argued that drug courts can do better, largely by focusing on what they are best at: monitoring treatment participation and providing access to resources. At the same time, drug court personnel should stop making treatment-related decisions, including whether particular forms of MAT are permissible and how long an individual can stay on MAT. If, however, drug courts insist on continuing to make treatment-related decisions, then they should at least include physicians, nurse practitioners, and physician assistants on their treatment teams. These medical professionals are more likely to accurately assess the risks and benefits of MAT relative to other team members lacking medical education.

GOAL 3

Methadone treatment becomes available through general practitioners after stabilization at opioid treatment programs

This is likely my most controversial goal. Yet if we examine the experience of the UK and France, there is little reason for the controversy.

In the UK, general practitioners can initiate methadone treatment for any patient who would benefit without special certification requirements or patient limits. In France, specialists initiate methadone treatment but then transfer patients to general practitioners once the patient is stabilized. In both nations, methadone is dispensed in community pharmacies with pharmacists playing an important role on the treatment team. The French example is likely to seem less extreme to many Americans than the UK example. Therefore, I posit that the French model is more achievable in the United States than the UK model, given our historical biases against expanding methadone treatment access—ironic since methadone treatment for opioid addiction began in the United States.

The benefits of permitting practitioners outside of OTPs to prescribe methadone to stabilized patients include the following: greater methadone treatment access for patients, particularly given the few OTP clinics in each state; integration of methadone treatment with other health services; and creating the perception of methadone treatment as part of mainstream medicine. Additionally, while many patients benefit from stepwise take-home limits where they "earn" take-home doses as stability increases, specific decisions regarding take-home allowances should be made by the physician and his or her team, with broad flexibility unimpeded by strict regulations. One of the most surprising results of my research is that many methadone treatment patients appreciate the accountability and responsibility associated with earning take-homes and the regular health service interaction afforded by daily dispensing (see chapter 4). But other patients are seriously inconvenienced by daily attendance requirements, especially when trying to maintain a job or take care of a family. Only flexibility in physician decision-making can address the variance in patient needs.

GOAL 4

Support groups for people undergoing MAT become accessible everywhere

There is no doubt that support groups, particularly twelve-step support groups, have helped millions of people in recovery around the world—so much so that some people become deeply offended if twelve-step groups are criticized at all. Nevertheless, one criticism has been repeated by many scholars, including me, yet largely ignored by local support groups: people undergoing MAT feel stigmatized when they discuss their treatment in twelve-step meetings.

Despite the stigmatization, many people undergoing MAT express a deep desire for concurrent twelve-step group participation and gratitude for the life skills that group membership has taught them. At the same time, they feel like hypocrites when compelled to hide one of the most effective tools they have used—medication—while being told during meetings that honesty is critical to recovery. Sometimes MAT stigmatization in twelve-step groups is so extreme that people are encouraged to stop MAT or to quit early, to their detriment. Ideally, twelve-step groups would be openly supportive of MAT, explicitly stating at meetings that MAT is an acceptable form of recovery and that it can be used in conjunction with twelve-step support. But numerous interviewees say that day is a long way off, especially for Narcotics Anonymous, in which stigma seems more salient than in Alcoholics Anonymous. Therefore, to meet the needs of people in recovery who desire the benefits of twelve-step peer support, new groups should be formed.

One such group, Medication-Assisted Recovery Anonymous (MARA), is a twelve-step group explicitly open to MAT. It is springing up in some cities around the nation but is still largely inaccessible to most Americans. Online versions may make it available in rural areas and small cities. Significantly more research is needed into the efficacy of groups like MARA, including online versions. Treatment centers can also initiate support groups that are peer-led and held on-site but that openly support MAT. The idea is not to displace existing support groups but to provide more peer support options to the many people who are tired of the pointless battle between twelve-step recovery approaches and MAT.

GOAL 5

Addiction treatment centers, whether inpatient, residential, or outpatient, offer a menu of treatment methods, including MAT

The Institute of Medicine and the Picker/Commonwealth Program for Patient-Centered Care have identified eight dimensions to person-centered care.[314,315] The first and possibly most important dimension is respect for patient preferences and values. Unfortunately, many SUD treatment centers today appear far from supportive of patient preferences and values. They typically offer one abstinence-only treatment track consisting entirely of detoxification, group counseling, and AA or NA, with little respect for individuals' unique recovery goals. Clients are given a preset program that they must follow or be asked to leave.

Theoretically, such one-track treatment centers would not be problematic if other multi-track treatment centers existed in the same area, allowing people to choose among a range of treatment centers. Yet small cities and rural areas rarely have treatment center variety. Even people living in urban areas may learn that what looks like a sea of treatment centers is a small puddle after eliminating those that do not take insurance or have months-long wait lists.

Therefore, the best health service approach is for every treatment center to offer a menu of treatment options, including all forms of MAT, individual counseling utilizing a variety of evidence-based methods, group counseling in which clients are matched to appropriate rather than arbitrary groups, and both spiritual and nonspiritual peer support. Furthermore, treatment centers should respect and support a wide range of goals, including complete abstinence, reduced drug use, and controlled drug use. It is not uncommon for people to fluctuate between different goals at different times. Obviously, each of these goals requires different outcome evaluation metrics, yet treatment centers primarily rely on the absence of drugs on a urine drug screen.

GOAL 6
Low-barrier buprenorphine treatment becomes widely available

Buprenorphine treatment is often "high barrier" in the United States, meaning that patients must meet a set of restrictive criteria to both begin and continue treatment (see chapter 3). To begin treatment, for example, they must demonstrate abstinence from all nonopioids, including marijuana, cocaine, alcohol, and benzodiazepines. To continue treatment, they must have negative urine drug screens for all drugs and opioids other than buprenorphine. If they miss more than a few doses, they are kicked out of treatment. Some treatment centers even require counseling or peer support group participation for buprenorphine access, even though the latest research suggests that not every person undergoing buprenorphine treatment benefits from additional psychosocial services.[23,316,317]

A low-barrier treatment approach largely eliminates these requirements, accepting patients under the theory that it is better to do some treatment than no treatment, even if the patient's participation is not ideal. It is a type of harm reduction. Relatedly, low-barrier treatment approaches often use a hub-and-spoke model, wherein the individual becomes a new patient immediately at the hub. After induction and stabilization, the individual is transferred to a spoke. The spoke is sometimes a higher-barrier treatment provider who would be uncomfortable treating someone who has not been stabilized.

The low-barrier buprenorphine treatment approach especially benefits people in vulnerable social situations, such as those experiencing homelessness or those who are uncertain about full recovery but want to start somewhere. It allows for treatment services to be established in resource-poor areas, including church basements and syringe exchange programs. Low-barrier treatment can also be combined with emergency department services for those who have recently overdosed. For example, following overdose reversal, the emergency department could provide up to three days' worth of buprenorphine, a legally permissive exception to the DATA-waiver requirement, after which the patient would immediately begin buprenorphine treatment in a low-barrier clinic. If only high-barrier clinics exist in the area, then the individual would likely wait weeks before beginning buprenorphine treatment—weeks during which another overdose is likely.

GOAL 7

People feel safe discussing their opioid problems, enabling them to seek treatment

I have arthritis. It is a chronic condition for which I take medication and watch my diet since some foods are linked to an inflammatory response. When I started exhibiting symptoms, I was confused about the symptoms' cause, but I felt no shame, even though at one point I was on crutches and pain prevented my participation in certain social events. I knew that I should seek treatment and immediately visited my primary care physician who then connected me to an orthopedic physician and ultimately to a rheumatologist. I had no trouble telling my family or friends. I was able to take some time off work to navigate the health services required to get me back on my feet.

If only people with opioid addiction felt the same level of comfort discussing their chronic health condition with others, enabling them to comfortably seek treatment resources without the fear of stigma or social backlash. Yet most instinctively hide their problem from family, friends, employers, and even health care providers. They fear being labeled as immoral or criminal. When the substance in question is itself illicit, such as heroin, then the stigma is heightened.

Destigmatization of any population is notoriously difficult, because stigma often builds on decades, if not centuries, of implicit and explicit derogatory beliefs about others, sometimes to the point that these beliefs become unconscious. Regular interaction with the stigmatized population can help decrease negative beliefs, as demonstrated by pharmacists in the UK and France who over time have come to see people with addiction less and less negatively. Courageous people in recovery sharing their stories with the public could slowly lead to a decrease in addiction-related stigma. But therein lies the rub: who wants to risk private and public backlash?

Decriminalization of drug possession could help disassociate addiction with criminality in the public's mind, but in most parts of the United States, we are a long way away from decriminalization. Nonprofit organizations or even the federal government could use billboards and other forms of public service announcements to share the fact that addiction is a health condition that cuts across race, income, gender, and other demographic variables rather than an indicator of morality. In the meantime, much more research evaluating the feasibility and efficacy of programs designed to destigmatize addiction is needed.

GOAL 8

The public has accurate knowledge about a full range of addiction treatments

Few studies have explored the public's knowledge about evidence-based treatments for opioid addiction, but existing data suggests that public knowledge is incomplete and heavily clouded by myths. In combination with low levels of education among health care providers about addiction medicine, it is no surprise that families of people in recovery feel lost in a tumultuous sea of treatment options. Family members have likely heard of AA, counseling, and rehab but may have little conception of what these recovery approaches entail. They are likely to have minimal knowledge about MAT.

Historically, any public service announcements related to drug use have primarily served a prevention aim—namely, warning the public of the danger of drugs. Public service announcements have rarely been used to educate people about treatment options. In other words, drug-related education has overwhelmingly focused on preventing people from developing addiction, leaving behind those who have already developed the condition, as if once you have addiction you are a lost cause. Researchers should seek to identify how best to educate the public about evidence-based treatment options. One such approach could include modifying existing public service announcements and education programs in schools so that people not only hear preventative messages but also learn what to do, or at least what reliable government resource to access, once an addiction has developed.

GOAL 9

Harm reduction becomes the norm

No one recovers from opioid addiction when they are dead. So, first and foremost, let's prevent overdose deaths by encouraging and training health care providers, emergency medical personnel, and police to distribute naloxone to people with opioid addiction and their family members. Additionally, naloxone should be available over the counter at a low cost in every pharmacy. Prisons and jails should provide naloxone upon release given the high overdose potential following incarceration.

Additionally, let's prevent unnecessary suffering from communicable diseases, such as HIV/AIDS and hepatitis C, among people who are actively using drugs. This requires widespread availability of syringes, such as through syringe exchange programs. Currently only some US cities operate syringe exchange programs, but these programs are far from adequate due to their low accessibility, stigmatization by the public and police, and lack of reliable funding. Ideally, syringe exchange programs would be complemented by federal and state law permitting community pharmacies to openly distribute and collect syringes, like in the UK. Such a law should go hand in hand with decriminalization of drug paraphernalia possession, which is often still illegal in areas where authorized syringe exchange programs operate. Finally, let's open supervised injection sites, especially given the growing evidence base of their benefits and minimal harms.

GOAL 10

Dual-diagnosis treatment becomes more widely available

Not everyone with an addiction has a co-occurring mental health disorder, such as depression, anxiety, or post-traumatic stress disorder. But study after study finds a high correlation between addiction and mental health disorders. Both similarly affect the brain, and the worsening of one disorder may negatively influence the other.

Ideally, treatment centers should offer services for both addiction and mental health. At the minimum, treatment providers of addiction should work collaboratively with offsite mental health treatment providers, and vice versa. Unfortunately, dual-diagnosis treatment today is rare, hampered by many of the same barriers that exist for addiction treatment, including stigma, lack of providers, and inadequate insurance reimbursement. Furthermore, addiction and mental health treatment providers may be deterred from collaboration by misunderstanding existing privacy laws, specifically 42 CFR 2 regulations, which require written consent from the patient for one treatment provider to share health records with another provider. Ideally, these regulations should be simplified, if not abandoned, in favor of HIPAA. At the minimum, treatment providers need better education about privacy law requirements so that they do not feel unnecessarily deterred from collaboration by misconceptions.

A Fictional Story of Jane Doe, September 2025, "Ideal City" in Anywhere, U.S.A.

A few months ago, Jane was prescribed oxycodone for low-back pain after all other treatments failed to give her any relief following a car accident. She never expected to become another person with opioid addiction. After a while, she took oxycodone not so much to treat back pain but rather to numb any unpleasant emotional sensations. She'd never really thought about it, but she'd probably been depressed for years. Oxycodone had become a bandage, albeit one that was causing more harm than healing.

When her boyfriend, Conor, yelled at her for not having the money to contribute to their rent after she secretly spent it all on oxycodone, and when her boss chewed her out for falling asleep during a work meeting, Jane took a hard look at her oxycodone use and decided to stop. But as soon as she tried to quit on her own, her depression worsened and she experienced flu-like symptoms, making her unable to concentrate on anything, least of all work.

"It's happened. I've developed opioid addiction," she told herself. It wasn't a comfortable fact to admit, but she knew it could happen to anyone. She knew she was not a bad person. She knew she needed medical help.

She sat her boyfriend down and told him about her problem. Fortunately, Conor had been educated about substance use disorders in public school and through public service announcements, so he knew addiction was not a choice even if Jane's first misuse of oxycodone was exactly that. He thanked God that Jane had not been arrested since drug possession and use had been recently decriminalized.

"I'll go call your primary care doctor," he said, "and get you an appointment for first thing tomorrow morning. In the meantime, contact your boss and tell her that you have a serious illness and need to take some time off work to recover. I'm sure your doctor will give you a note tomorrow." Conor then called Jane's primary care physician's office and asked for an appointment for the next day. When the receptionist asked what the problem was, he said his girlfriend had opioid addiction. The receptionist did not act surprised or judgmental while scheduling Jane for the following morning.

The next day, Conor and Jane attended the primary care appointment together. Jane was forthcoming about how she started misusing oxycodone. She had expected the conversation to be embarrassing, especially given that this primary care physician was the same one who had prescribed the oxycodone to begin with for her low-back pain. But the physician seemed completely unfazed. He asked Jane if she'd thought about treatment options and whether she had any preferences. He also asked about her goals.

Jane said she'd like to quit oxycodone entirely and try buprenorphine as a recovery tool. She said she was not sure she could handle the full detoxification required for extended-release naltrexone, at least not yet, even though she would eventually like to be opioid-free. The physician responded that there was no rush to be opioid-free; what was most important was that she was starting her recovery. They also discussed methadone as an option, but Jane decided she did not want to travel to a methadone clinic daily, even though the primary care physician could eventually prescribe the methadone and have it dispensed at the local pharmacy after stabilization.

The physician asked whether Jane would like to participate in counseling and peer support groups as well, since psychosocial support could help her depression symptoms and keep her focused on her recovery. Jane agreed that the counseling would likely be beneficial, but she said she'd only be in a peer support group that is supportive of buprenorphine treatment. The physician nodded and introduced Jane to his case manager, Terry. Without needing any extra paperwork, Terry made some phone calls to local addiction counselors. A few minutes later, Terry informed Jane that a counselor in a mental health clinic would see her the following week. Terry also provided brochures for a range of local peer support groups, including spiritual and nonspiritual ones, and ones that explicitly accepted people utilizing MAT.

The physician then conducted a comprehensive physical and mental health examination, after which he explained the risks and benefits of buprenorphine treatment. Jane decided she wanted to move forward with it, so the physician administered the first dose of buprenorphine directly. A nurse kept Jane under observation for an hour to make sure no unexpected side effects occurred. None did. The physician then returned and handed Jane a prescription for a month's medication supply, telling her to come in for a follow-up appointment in one month but to contact the office earlier if needed.

Jane and Conor drove to the local pharmacy where they picked up the buprenorphine prescription immediately as no prior insurance authorization was required and the pharmacy was fully stocked. The pharmacist was friendly and nonjudgmental, asking Jane if she had any questions or concerns about buprenorphine. Conor bought some naloxone over the counter while Jane waited for her prescription to be filled, feeling for the first time in months like everything was going to be okay.

Acknowledgments

There are many people who contributed to this book, such as through assisting me with my research, providing me with endless streams of encouragement, and providing suggestions on how to improve the readability of what could otherwise be a dense topic. Most importantly, thank you to every person I interviewed. Even though I am keeping your identity confidential, please know that this book would not exist without the courage you demonstrated in sharing your story.

A big thank you to Robin Coleman, my editor at Johns Hopkins University Press, for his many hours of hard work and support. I especially appreciate you pushing me to write a book not just for researchers and health practitioners but also for lay readers and anyone affected by or interested in the opioid overdose crisis.

I probably would not have tried to publish this book without encouragement from Professor Jody Lynee Madeira at the Indiana University Maurer School of Law, who has served as both my PhD supervisor and mentor. Thank you for urging me to update and transform my dissertation for a broader audience, as well as for the many detailed suggestions you provided along the way for improving the manuscript.

I also wish to thank Professor Dennis Watson at the University of Illinois at Chicago, Professor Christopher Harle at the University of Florida, and Professor Kosali Simon at the Indiana University School of Public Health and Environmental Affairs, each of whom taught me research methodology for health services and health policy, including during my postdoctoral fellowship. Thank you to Matthew James Capone, Olivia Randall-Kosich, and Rachel Totaram for their assistance with data collection and research analysis. I also appreciate the numerous educational conversations I have had with three passionate addiction psychiatrists: Dr. Andrew Chambers, Dr. Nishanie

Gunawardane, and Dr. Camila Arnaudo. Thank you to Chris Abert of the Indiana Recovery Alliance and Justin Kunzelman of Rebel Recovery for teaching me about harm reduction principles and allowing me to serve on your organizations' boards.

Finally, thank you to my loving family, Margaret Andraka, Bohdan Andraka, Natalia Andraka, and Tomasz Andraka, for their encouragement along this journey. Thank you to my children, Magdalena Christou and Nikolaos Christou, for opening my heart and reminding me of my priorities. And last but not least, thank you to my husband, Alexander Christou, to whom I dedicate this book, for always believing in me and for putting up with many late nights while I finalized a book that I hope will change many lives.

References

1. Dube SR, Felitti VJ, Dong M, Chapman DP, Giles WH, Anda RF. Childhood abuse, neglect, and household dysfunction and the risk of illicit drug use: the adverse childhood experiences study. *Pediatrics*. 2003;111(3): 564–572. http://pediatrics.aappublications.org/content/pediatrics/111/3/564.full.pdf. Accessed February 2, 2018.
2. Felitti VJ, Anda RF, Nordenberg D, et al. Relationship of childhood abuse and household dysfunction to many of the leading causes of death in adults: the adverse childhood experiences (ACE) study. *Am J Prev Med*. 1998;14(4):245–258. In: https://www.cambridgema.gov/CDD/Projects/Planning/~/media/328D3B716A24449D8504357BD3865949.ashx. Accessed January 25, 2019.
3. *The Role of Adverse Childhood Experiences in Substance Misuse and Related Behavioral Health Problems*. SAMHSA's Center for the Application of Prevention Technologies; 2018. https://www.cambridgema.gov/CDD/Projects/Planning/~/media/328D3B716A24449D8504357BD3865949.ashx. Accessed January 25, 2019.
4. *Comorbidity: Addiction & Other Mental Illnesses*. NIDA Research Report Series. NIH Publication Number 10-5771. North Bethesda, MD: National Institutes of Health, National Institute on Drug Abuse; 2010. https://www.drugabuse.gov/sites/default/files/rrcomorbidity.pdf. Accessed February 6, 2018.
5. Mandavia A, Robinson GGN, Bradley B, Ressler KJ, Powers A. Exposure to childhood abuse and later substance use: indirect effects of emotion dysregulation and exposure to trauma. *J Trauma*. 2016;29(5):422–429. doi:10.1002/jts.22131.
6. Mirhashem R, Allen HC, Adams ZW, Van Stolk-Cooke K, Legrand A, Price M. The intervening role of urgency on the association between childhood maltreatment, PTSD, and substance-related problems. *Addict Behav*. 2017;69:98–103. doi:10.1016/j.addbeh.2017.02.012.
7. Centers for Disease Control & Prevention. Wide-ranging online data for epidemiologic research (WONDER). https://wonder.cdc.gov/. Published 2016. Accessed December 1, 2017.
8. Opioid overdose crisis. National Institute on Drug Abuse website. https://www.drugabuse.gov/drugs-abuse/opioids/opioid-overdose-crisis. Updated January 2019. Accessed August 10, 2019.
9. Ciccarone D. The triple wave epidemic: supply and demand drivers of the US opioid overdose crisis. *Int J Drug Policy*. Published online February 1, 2019. doi:10.1016/j.drugpo.2019.01.010.

10. Ghertner R, Groves L. *The Opioid Crisis and Economic Opportunity: Geographic and Economic Trends*. ASPE Research Brief. Washington, DC: US Department of Health and Human Services, Office of the Assistant Secretary for Planning and Evaluation; 2018. https://aspe.hhs.gov/system/files/pdf/259261/ASPEEconomicOpportunityOpioidCrisis.pdf. Accessed January 25, 2019.
11. Addiction science. National Institute on Drug Abuse website. https://www.drugabuse.gov/related-topics/addiction-science. Updated July 2015. Accessed August 10, 2019.
12. Whelan PJ, Remski K. Buprenorphine vs methadone treatment: a review of evidence in both developed and developing worlds. *J Neurosci Rural Pract*. 2012;3(1):45–50. doi:10.4103/0976-3147.91934.
13. Nielsen S, Larance B, Lintzeris N. Opioid agonist treatment for patients with dependence on prescription opioids. *J Am Med Assoc*. 2017;317(9): 967–968. doi:10.1001/jama.2017.0001.
14. Larochelle MR, Bernson D, Land T, et al. Medication for opioid use disorder after nonfatal opioid overdose and association with mortality: a cohort study. *Ann Intern Med*. 2018;169(3):137–145. doi:10.7326/M17-3107.
15. Larney S. Does opioid substitution treatment in prisons reduce injecting-related HIV risk behaviours? A systematic review. *Addiction*. 2010;105(2): 216–223. doi:10.1111/j.1360-0443.2009.02826.x.
16. Hedrich D, Alves P, Farrell M, Stöver H, Møller L, Mayet S. The effectiveness of opioid maintenance treatment in prison settings: a systematic review. *Addiction*. 2012;107(3):501–517. doi:10.1111/j.1360-0443.2011.03676.x.
17. Lappalainen L, Nolan S, Dobrer S, et al. Dose-response relationship between methadone dose and adherence to antiretroviral therapy among HIV-positive persons who use illicit opioids. *Addiction*. 2015;110(8): 1330–1339. doi:10.1111/add.12970.
18. Magura S, Lee JD, Hershberger J, et al. Buprenorphine and methadone maintenance in jail and post-release: a randomized clinical trial. *Drug Alcohol Depend*. 2009;99(1–3):222–230 doi:10.1016/j.drugalcdep.2008.08.006.
19. Bart G. Maintenance medication for opiate addiction: the foundation of recovery. *J Addict Dis*. 2012;31(3):207–225. doi:10.1080/10550887.2012.694598.
20. Roman PM, Abraham AJ, Knudsen HK. Using medication-assisted treatment for substance use disorders: evidence of barriers and facilitators of implementation. *Addict Behav*. 2011;36(6):584–589. doi:10.1016/j.addbeh.2011.01.032.
21. Abraham AJ, Knudsen HK, Rieckmann T, Roman PM. Disparities in access to physicians and medications for the treatment of substance use

disorders between publicly and privately funded treatment programs in the United States. *J Stud Alcohol Drugs*. 2013;74(2):258–265. doi:10.15288/jsad.2013.74.258.

22. Potter JS, Marino EN, Hillhouse MP, et al. Buprenorphine/naloxone and methadone maintenance treatment outcomes for opioid analgesic, heroin, and combined users: findings from starting treatment with agonist replacement therapies (START). *J Stud Alcohol Drugs*. 2013;74(4):605–613.
23. Substance Abuse and Mental Health Services Administration. *TIP 63: Medications for Opioid Use Disorder for Healthcare and Addiction Professionals, Policymakers, Patients, and Families*. HHS Publication No. (SMA) 19-5063FULLDOC. Rockville, MD: SAMHSA; 2018. https://store.samhsa.gov/product/TIP-63-Medications-for-Opioid-Use-Disorder-Full-Document-Including-Executive-Summary-and-Parts-1-5-/SMA18-5063FULLDOC. Accessed July 9, 2018.
24. World Health Organization, United Nations Office on Drugs and Crime, Joint United Nations Programme on HIV/AIDS. *Substitution Maintenance Therapy in the Management of Opioid Dependence and HIV/AIDS Prevention*. WHO/UNODC/UNAIDS position paper. Geneva, Switzerland: WHO; 2004. https://www.who.int/substance_abuse/publications/en/PositionPaper_English.pdf. Accessed August 10, 2019.
25. Sharma A, O'Grady KE, Kelly SM, Gryczynski J, Mitchell SG, Schwartz RP. Pharmacotherapy for opioid dependence in jails and prisons: research review update and future directions. *Subst Abuse Rehabil*. 2016;7:27–40. doi:10.2147/SAR.S81602.
26. Remarks from FDA Commissioner Scott Gottlieb, M.D., as prepared for oral testimony before the House Committee on Energy and Commerce Hearing, "Federal Efforts to Combat the Opioid Crisis: A Status Update on CARA and Other Initiatives" [news release]. Silver Spring, MD: Food and Drug Administration; October 25, 2017. https://www.fda.gov/NewsEvents/Newsroom/PressAnnouncements/ucm582031.htm. Accessed August 10, 2019.
27. US Department of Health and Human Services (HHS), Office of the Surgeon General. *Facing Addiction in America: The Surgeon General's Spotlight on Opioids*. Washington, DC: HHS; September 2018. https://addiction.surgeongeneral.gov/sites/default/files/Spotlight-on-Opioids_09192018.pdf. Accessed January 16, 2019.
28. Leshner AI, Mancher M, eds. *Medications for Opioid Use Disorder Save Lives*. Washington, DC: National Academies Press; 2019. doi:10.17226/25310.
29. Lopez G. 2016 opioid overdoses killed more Americans than Iraq and Vietnam. *Vox*. July 7, 2017. www.vox.com/policy-and-politics/2017/7/7/15925488/opioid-epidemic-deaths-2016. Accessed August 10, 2019.
30. Dowell D, Arias E, Kochanek K, et al. Contribution of opioid-involved poisoning to the change in life expectancy in the United States, 2000–2015.

JAMA. 2017;318(11):1065–1067. doi:10.1001/JAMA.2017.9308.

31. Salihu HM, Wilson RE, King LM, Marty PJ, Whiteman VE. Socio-ecological model as a framework for overcoming barriers and challenges in randomized control trials in minority and underserved communities. *Int J MCH AIDS*. 2015;3(1):85–95. http://www.ncbi.nlm.nih.gov/pubmed/27621990. Accessed April 27, 2018.
32. Montano DE, Kasprzyk D. Theory of reasoned action, theory of planned behavior, and the integrated behavioral model. In: Glanz K, Rimer BK, Viswanath K, eds. *Health Behavior and Health Education: Theory, Research, and Practice*. 4th ed. San Francisco, CA: Jossey-Bass; 2008:67–96.
33. Waldorf D, Orlick M, Reinarman C. *Morphine Maintenance: The Shreveport Clinic 1919–1923*. Washington, DC: Drug Abuse Council; 1974.
34. *Webb v United States*, 249 US 96 (1919).
35. White WL. *Slaying the Dragon: The History of Addiction Treatment & Recovery in America*. Bloomington, IL: Chestnut; 1998.
36. Musto D, Ramos M. Notes on American history: a follow-up study of the New Haven morphine maintenance clinic of 1920. *N Engl J Med*. 1981; 304(18):1071–1077.
37. America's first drug-treatment prison revisited [transcript]. *All Things Considered*. National Public Radio. November 1, 2008. https://www.npr.org/templates/story/story.php?storyId=96437766. Accessed August 10, 2019.
38. Conversation with Jerome H. Jaffe. *Addiction*. 1999;94(1):13–30. doi:10.1080/09652149934143.
39. Addiction research: Jerome Jaffe, interviewed by Nancy Campbell for the Oral History of Substance Abuse Research project [transcript]. Published 1969. http://www.williamwhitepapers.com/pr/2013 Dr. Jerome Jaffe.pdf. Accessed January 26, 2019.
40. Courtwright DT. *Dark Paradise: A History of Opiate Addiction*. Cambridge, MA: Harvard University Press; 2001.
41. Campbell N, Olsen JP, Walden L. *The Narcotic Farm: The Rise and Fall of America's First Prison for Drug Addicts*. New York, NY: Harry N Abrams Inc; 2008.
42. Massing M. *The Fix*. Los Angeles: University of California Press; 1998.
43. Clark C. *The Recovery Revolution: The Battle over Addiction Treatment in the United States*. New York, NY: Columbia University Press; 2017.
44. Doberteen L. *Orange Handcuffs, Part of an (In)Complete Breakfast: Methadone's Failure to Address Structural Inequalities in the Civil Rights Era* [thesis]. New York, NY: Columbia University; 2015.
45. Shuster A. GI heroin addiction epidemic in Vietnam. *New York Times*. May 16, 1971. http://www.nytimes.com/1971/05/16/archives/gi-heroin-addiction-epidemic-in-vietnam-gi-heroin-addiction-is.html. Accessed August 10, 2019.

46. Drug wars: interview with Dr. Jerome Jaffe [edited transcript]. *Frontline*. PBS; 2000. https://www.pbs.org/wgbh/pages/frontline/shows/drugs/interviews/jaffe.html. Accessed February 8, 2018.
47. Jaffe JH, O'Keeffe C. From morphine clinics to buprenorphine: regulating opioid agonist treatment of addiction in the United States. *Drug Alcohol Depend*. 2003;70(2):S3–S11. doi:10.1016/S0376-8716(03)00055-3.
48. Reuter P. Why has US drug policy changed so little over 30 years? *Crime and Justice*. 2013;42(1):75–140. doi:10.1086/670818.
49. Cherkis J. Nancy Reagan's legacy includes support of abusive drug treatment for teens. *Huffington Post*. March 7, 2016. https://www.huffingtonpost.com/entry/nancy-reagan-drug-treatment-straight-inc_us_56ddda84e4b03a405679693e. Accessed August 10, 2019.
50. Drucker E. Failed drug policies in the United States and the future of AIDS: a perfect storm. *J Public Heal Policy*. 2012;33(3):309–316. http://www.jstor.org/stable/pdf/23253451.pdf. Accessed February 8, 2018.
51. Kohn H. Cowboy in the capital: drug czar Bill Bennett. *Rolling Stone*. November 2, 1989. https://www.rollingstone.com/politics/politics-news/cowboy-in-the-capital-drug-czar-bill-bennett-45472/. Accessed January 26, 2019.
52. Bennett W. *National Drug Control Strategy*. Washington, DC: Office of National Drug Control Policy; September 1989. https://www.ncjrs.gov/pdffiles1/ondcp/119466.pdf. Accessed January 26, 2019.
53. Bennett W, Walters JP. Bring back the war on drugs. *Boston Globe*. September 9, 2015. https://www.hudson.org/research/11585-bring-back-the-war-on-drugs. Accessed August 10, 2019.
54. Burns RM, Pacula RL, Bauhoff S, et al. Policies related to opioid agonist therapy for opioid use disorders: the evolution of state policies from 2004 to 2013. *Subst Abus*. 2016;37(1):63–69. doi:10.1080/08897077.2015.1080208.
55. Campbell ND, Lovell AM. The history of the development of buprenorphine as an addiction therapeutic. *Ann N Y Acad Sci*. 2012;1248(1):124–139. doi:10.1111/j.1749-6632.2011.06352.x.
56. Harper J. To grow market share, a drugmaker pitches its product to judges. *Shots: Health News from NPR*. National Public Radio. August 3, 2017. https://www.npr.org/sections/health-shots/2017/08/03/540029500/to-grow-market-share-a-drugmaker-pitches-its-product-to-judges. Accessed August 10, 2019.
57. Jackson H, Mandell K, Johnson K, Chatterjee D, Vanness DJ. Cost-effectiveness of injectable extended-release naltrexone compared with methadone maintenance and buprenorphine maintenance treatment for opioid dependence. *Subst Abus*. 2015;36(2):226–231. doi:10.1080/08897077.2015.1010031.
58. Lee JD, Nunes EV, Novo P, et al. Comparative effectiveness of extended-

release naltrexone versus buprenorphine-naloxone for opioid relapse prevention (X:BOT): a multicentre, open-label, randomised controlled trial. *Lancet*. 2018;391(10118):309–318. doi:10.1016/S0140-6736(17)32812-X.

59. Tanum L, Solli KK, Latif Z-H, et al. The effectiveness of injectable extended-release naltrexone vs daily buprenorphine-naloxone for opioid dependence. *JAMA Psychiatry*. 2017;74(12):1197–1205. doi:10.1001/jamapsychiatry.2017.3206.
60. Morgan JR, Schackman BR, Leff JA, Linas BP, Walley AY. Injectable naltrexone, oral naltrexone, and buprenorphine utilization and discontinuation among individuals treated for opioid use disorder in a United States commercially insured population. *J Subst Abuse Treat*. 2018;85:90–96. doi:10.1016/j.jsat.2017.07.001.
61. Yokell MA, Zaller ND, Green TC, Rich JD. Buprenorphine and buprenorphine/naloxone diversion, misuse, and illicit use: an international review. *Curr Drug Abus Rev*. 2011;4(1):28–41. https://www-ncbi-nlm-nih-gov.proxy.medlib.uits.iu.edu/pmc/articles/PMC3154701/pdf/nihms314965.pdf. Accessed October 24, 2017.
62. Khanna IK, Pillarisetti S. Buprenorphine: an attractive opioid with underutilized potential in treatment of chronic pain. *J Pain Res*. 2015;8:859–870. doi:10.2147/JPR.S85951.
63. Gaebel W, Zäske H, Cleveland HR, et al. Measuring the stigma of psychiatry and psychiatrists: development of a questionnaire. *Eur Arch Psychiatry Clin Neurosci*. 2011;261(Suppl 2):S119–123. doi:10.1007/s00406-011-0252-0.
64. Fatséas M, Auriacombe M. Why buprenorphine is so successful in treating opiate addiction in France. *Curr Psychiatry Rep*. 2007;9(5):358–364. doi:10.1007/s11920-007-0046-2.
65. Schedules of controlled substances: Rescheduling of buprenorphine from Schedule V to Schedule III. *Fed. Regist*. 2002;67(194):62354–62370. To be codified at 21 CFR §1308. https://www.govinfo.gov/content/pkg/FR-2002-10-07/pdf/02-25293.pdf. Accessed August 10, 2019.
66. Facher L. Nearly all doctors can freely prescribe opioids. Now a new movement aims to vastly deregulate an addiction treatment. *STAT News*. April 30, 2019. https://www.statnews.com/2019/04/30/loosen-restrictions-on-prescribing-buprenorphine-addiction-treatment. Accessed August 10, 2019.
67. Andraka-Christou B. America needs the TREAT Act: expanding access to effective medication for treating addiction. *Health Matrix Clevel*. 2016;26:309–362.
68. Pub L No. 109-56, 119 Stat 591 (2005). https://www.congress.gov/109/plaws/publ56/PLAW-109publ56.pdf. Accessed August 10, 2019.
69. Office of National Drug Control Policy Reauthorization Act of 2006,

Pub L No. 109-469, 120 Stat 3502. https://www.congress.gov/109/plaws/publ469/PLAW-109publ469.htm. Accessed August 10, 2019.

70. Statement of Senator Orrin Hatch regarding the Office of National Drug Control Policy Reauthorization Act of 2006. *Cong Rec Sen.* 2006;152(135): S11703–S11706.
71. Vestal C. Waiting lists grow for medicine to fight opioid addiction. *Huffington Post*. February 11, 2016. http://www.huffingtonpost.com/entry/opioid-addiction-treatment_us_56bcb1a5e4b08ffac1241b63. Accessed August 10, 2019.
72. Schuman-Olivier Z, Connery H, Griffin ML, et al. Clinician beliefs and attitudes about buprenorphine/naloxone diversion. *Am J Addict.* 2013; 22(6):574–580. doi:10.1111/j.1521-0391.2013.12024.x.
73. Johanson CE, Arfken CL, di Menza S, Schuster CR. Diversion and abuse of buprenorphine: findings from national surveys of treatment patients and physicians. *Drug Alcohol Depend.* 2012;120(1–3):190–195. doi:10.1016/j.drugalcdep.2011.07.019.
74. Genberg BL, Gillespie M, Schuster CR, et al. Prevalence and correlates of street-obtained buprenorphine use among current and former injectors in Baltimore, Maryland. *Addict Behav.* 2013;38(12):2868–2873. doi:10.1016/j.addbeh.2013.08.008.
75. Office Based Opioid Treatment Programs, S 398, 120th Gen Assem, 2nd Sess (In 2018). https://iga.in.gov/legislative/2018/bills/senate/398#document-dc532596. Accessed February 8, 2018.
76. Subramaniam G, Levy S, Sullivan MA. *PCSS Guidance Topic: Treatment of Opioid-Dependent Adolescents and Young Adults Using Sublingual Buprenorphine.* East Providence, RI: Providers' Clinical Support System; 2013. https://30qkon2g8eif8wrj03zeh041-wpengine.netdna-ssl.com/wp-content/uploads/2014/03/PCSS-MATGuidanceTreatmentofOpioidDependantAdolescent-buprenorphine.SubramaniamLevy1.pdf. Accessed October 27, 2018.
77. Trial AR, Woody GE, Poole SA, et al. Extended vs short-term buprenorphine-naloxone for treatment of opioid-addicted youth: a randomized trial. *JAMA.* 2008;300(17):2003–2011.
78. Harper J. A drugmaker tries to cash in on the opioid epidemic, one state law at a time. *Shots: Health News from NPR.* National Public Radio. June 12, 2017.
79. Schwarz A. Michael Botticelli is a drug czar who knows addiction firsthand. *New York Times.* April 25, 2015. https://www.nytimes.com/2015/04/26/us/michael-botticelli-is-a-drug-czar-who-knows-addiction-firsthand.html. Accessed August 10, 2019.
80. Botticelli M. Remarks at: The Road Back from the Opioid Crisis: Lessons for State Leadership; September 17, 2015; Arlington, VA. https://obamawhitehouse.archives.gov/the-press-office/2015/09/17

/remarks-ondcp-director-michael-botticelli. Accessed February 8, 2018.
81. Volkow ND, Frieden TR, Hyde PS, Cha SS. Medication-assisted therapies—tackling the opioid-overdose epidemic. *N Engl J Med.* 2014; 370(22):2063–2066. doi:10.1056/NEJMp1402780.
82. Brooklyn JR, Sigmon SC. Vermont hub-and-spoke model of care for opioid use disorder: development, implementation, and impact. *J Addict Med.* 2017;11(4):286–292. doi:10.1097/ADM.0000000000000310.
83. Comprehensive Addiction and Recovery Act, S 524, 114th Cong (2016). https://www.congress.gov/bill/114th-congress/senate-bill/524/text. Accessed February 8, 2018.
84. Fiscella K, Wakeman SE, Beletsky L. Buprenorphine deregulation and mainstreaming treatment for opioid use disorder: X the X waiver. *JAMA Psychiatry.* 2019;76(3):229–230. doi:10.1001/jamapsychiatry.2018.3685.
85. 21st Century Cures Act, HR 34, 114th Cong (2016). https://www.congress.gov/bill/114th-congress/house-bill/34/. Accessed February 8, 2018.
86. Trump budget doubles down on drug war [news release]. New York, NY: Drug Policy Alliance; February 12, 2018. http://www.drugpolicy.org/press-release/2018/02/trump-budget-doubles-down-drug-war. Accessed August 10, 2019.
87. The federal drug control budget: new rhetoric, same failed drug war [fact sheet]. New York, NY: Drug Policy Alliance; February 2015. https://www.drugpolicy.org/sites/default/files/DPA_Fact_sheet_Drug_War_Budget_Feb2015.pdf. Accessed August 10, 2019.
88. Christie C, Baker C, Cooper R, Kennedy PJ, Madras B, Bondi P. The president's commission on combating drug addiction and the opioid crisis. https://www.whitehouse.gov/sites/whitehouse.gov/files/images/Final_Report_Draft_11-15-2017.pdf. Published November 2017. Accessed February 8, 2018.
89. Lopez G. Trump just signed a bipartisan bill to confront the opioid epidemic. *Vox.* October 24, 2018. https://www.vox.com/policy-and-politics/2018/9/28/17913938/trump-opioid-epidemic-congress-support-act-bill-law. Accessed August 10, 2019.
90. President Donald J. Trump is taking action on drug addiction and the opioid crisis [fact sheet]. Washington, DC: White House Briefings & Statements; October 26, 2017. https://www.whitehouse.gov/briefings-statements/president-donald-j-trump-taking-action-drug-addiction-opioid-crisis/. Accessed February 8, 2018.
91. Opioid treatment program directory. Substance Abuse and Mental Health Services Administration website. https://dpt2.samhsa.gov/treatment/directory.aspx. Accessed June 3, 2018.
92. Mattick RP, Breen C, Kimber J, Davoli M. Methadone maintenance therapy versus no opioid replacement therapy for opioid dependence.

Cochrane Database Syst Rev. 2009;(3):CD002209. doi:10.1002/14651858.CD002209.pub2.

93. Rosenblatt RA, Andrilla CHA, Catlin M, Larson EH. Geographic and specialty distribution of US physicians trained to treat opioid use disorder. *Ann Fam Med*. 2015;13(1):23–26. doi:10.1370/afm.1735.
94. Hansen H, Siegel C, Wanderling J, DiRocco D. Buprenorphine and methadone treatment for opioid dependence by income, ethnicity and race of neighborhoods in New York City. *Drug Alcohol Depend*. 2016;164:14–21. doi:10.1016/j.drugalcdep.2016.03.028.
95. Lagisetty PA, Ross R, Bohnert A, Clay M, Maust DT. Buprenorphine treatment divide by race/ethnicity and payment. *JAMA Psychiatry*. Published online May 8, 2019. doi:10.1001/jamapsychiatry.2019.0876.
96. Stein BD, Dick AW, Sorbero M, et al. A population-based examination of trends and disparities in medication treatment for opioid use disorders among Medicaid enrollees. *Subst Abus*. 2018;39(4):419–425. doi:10.1080/08897077.2018.1449166.
97. Substance Abuse and Mental Health Services Administration. *National Survey of Substance Abuse Treatment Services (N-SSATS): 2013. Data on Substance Abuse Treatment Facilities*. BHSIS Series S-73, HHS Publication No. (SMA) 14-489. Rockville, MD: SAMHSA; 2014. https://www.samhsa.gov/data/sites/default/files/2013_N-SSATS/2013_N-SSATS_National_Survey_of_Substance_Abuse_Treatment_Services.pdf. Accessed February 8, 2018.
98. Wu L-T, Zhu H, Swartz MS. Treatment utilization among persons with opioid use disorder in the United States. *Drug Alcohol Depend*. 2016;169:117–127. doi:10.1016/j.drugalcdep.2016.10.015.
99. West SL, O'Neal KK. Project D.A.R.E. outcome effectiveness revisited. *Am J Public Health*. 2004;94(6):1027–1029.
100. Pagano ME, White WL, Kelly JF, Stout RL, Carter RR, Tonigan JS. The 10-year course of AA participation and long-term outcomes: a follow-up study of outpatient subjects in Project MATCH. *Subst Abus*. 2013;34(1):51–59. doi:10.1080/08897077.2012.691450.
101. Nielsen S, Larance B, Degenhardt L, Gowing L, Kehler C, Lintzeris N. Opioid agonist treatment for pharmaceutical opioid dependent people. *Cochrane Database Syst Rev*. 2016;(5):CD011117. doi:10.1002/14651858.CD011117.pub2.
102. Saloner B, Karthikeyan S, RC D, et al. Changes in substance abuse treatment use among individuals with opioid use disorders in the United States, 2004–2013. *JAMA*. 2015;314(14):1515–1517. doi:10.1001/jama.2015.10345.
103. Roman PM, Johnson JA. *National Treatment Center Study Summary Report: Private Treatment Centers*. Athens, GA: Institute for Behavioral Research;

2004. http://ntcs.uga.edu/reports/NTCS summary reports/NTCS Report No. 7.pdf. Accessed February 21, 2018.

104. Andraka-Christou B. What is treatment for opioid addiction in problem-solving courts? A study of 20 Indiana drug & veterans courts. *Stanford J Civ Rights Civ Lib*. 2017;13(2):189–254.

105. Substance abuse probation. 204 Pennsylvania Administrative Code §89.293. https://www.padisciplinaryboard.org/for-attorneys/rules/rule/7/disciplinary-board-rules-and-procedures. Accessed August 10, 2019.

106. Berge K, Sepalla M, Schipper A. Chemical dependency and the physician. *Mayo Clin Proc*. 2009;84(7):625–631. https://www.ncbi.nlm.nih.gov/pmc/articles/PMC2704134/. Accessed August 10, 2019.

107. Walters GD. Twelve reasons why we need to find alternatives to Alcoholics Anonymous. *Addict Disord Their Treat*. 2002;1(2):53–59. https://journals.lww.com/addictiondisorders/Abstract/2002/06000/Twelve_Reasons_Why_We_Need_to_Find_Alternatives_to.3.aspx. Accessed August 10, 2019.

108. Travis T. *The Language of the Heart: A Cultural History of the Recovery Movement from Alcoholics Anonymous to Oprah Winfrey*. Chapel Hill: University of North Carolina Press; 2009.

109. Whelan PJP, Marshall EJ, Ball DM, Humphreys K. The role of AA sponsors: a pilot study. *Alcohol Alcohol*. 2009;44(4):416–422. doi:10.1093/alcalc/agp014.

110. The twelve steps of Alcoholics Anonymous [service material]. New York, NY: Alcoholics Anonymous Publishing; 1981. https://www.aa.org/assets/en_US/smf-121_en.pdf. Updated August 2016. Accessed on August 10, 2019.

111. Tournier RE. Alcoholics Anonymous as treatment and as ideology. *J Stud Alcohol*. 1979;40(3):230–239.

112. Estimates of AA groups and members as of January 1, 2017 [service material]. New York, NY: AA World Services; 2017. https://www.aa.org/assets/en_US/smf-53_en.pdf. Updated March 2019. Accessed April 10, 2018.

113. Humphreys K, Wing S, McCarty D, et al. Self-help organizations for alcohol and drug problems: toward evidence-based practice and policy. *J Subst Abuse Treat*. 2004;26(3):151–158. doi:10.1016/S0740-5472(03)00212-5.

114. Kessler R, Mickelson K, Zhao S. Patterns and correlates of self-help group membership in the United States. *Soc Policy*. 1997;27(3):27–46. http://citeseerx.ist.psu.edu/viewdoc/download?doi=10.1.1.372.1885&rep=rep1&type=pdf. Accessed August 10, 2019.

115. Humphreys K. *Circles of Recovery: Self-Help Organizations for Addictions*. Cambridge, UK: Cambridge University Press; 2004.

116. Miller M. The relevance of twelve-step recovery in 21st century addiction medicine. *ASAM Magazine* [blog]. American Society of Addiction Medicine website. February 13, 2015.
117. Knudsen HK, Abraham AJ, Oser CB. *National Treatment Center Study Project Report, Barriers to the Adoption of Pharmacotherapies in Publicly Funded Substance Abuse Treatment: Policy Barriers and Access to Physicians*. Athens, GA: Institute for Behavioral Research; 2011. http://ntcs.uga.edu/reports/Medications in Publicly Funded Treatment.pdf. Accessed February 21, 2018.
118. Rieckmann TR, Kovas AE, McFarland BH, Abraham AJ. Counselor attitudes toward the use of buprenorphine in substance abuse treatment: a multi-level modeling approach. *J Subst Abuse Treat.* 2011;41(4):374–385. doi:10.1016/j.jsat.2011.05.005.
119. Knudsen HK, Ducharme LJ, Roman PM, Link T. Buprenorphine diffusion: the attitudes of substance abuse treatment counselors. *J Subst Abuse Treat.* 2005;29(2):95–106. doi:10.1016/j.jsat.2005.05.002.
120. Magura S, Rosenblum A. Leaving methadone treatment: lessons learned, lessons forgotten, lessons ignored. *Mt Sinai J Med.* 2001;68(1):62–74. http://www.ncbi.nlm.nih.gov/pubmed/11135508. Accessed February 9, 2018.
121. Clausen T, Anchersen K, Waal H. Mortality prior to, during and after opioid maintenance treatment (OMT): a national prospective cross-registry study. *Drug Alcohol Depend.* 2008;94(1–3):151–157. doi:10.1016/j.drugalcdep.2007.11.003.
122. Gilman SM, Dermatis H, Galanter M. Methadone Anonymous: a 12-step program for methadone maintained heroin addicts. *Subst Abus.* 2001; 22(4):247–256. doi:10.1080/08897070109511466.
123. Narcotics Anonymous and persons receiving medication-assisted treatment [pamphlet]. Chatsworth, CA: NA World Services Inc.; 2016. https://www.na.org/admin/include/spaw2/uploads/pdf/pr/2306_NA_PRMAT_1021.pdf. Accessed August 10, 2019.
124. Regarding methadone and other drug replacement programs. World Service Board of Trustees Bulletin #29. Van Nuys, CA: Narcotics Anonymous World Services; 1996. https://www.na.org/?ID=bulletins-bull29. Accessed February 9, 2018.
125. Suzuki J, Dodds T. Clinician recommendation of 12-step meeting attendance and discussion regarding disclosure of buprenorphine use among patients in office-based opioid treatment. *Subst Abus.* 2016;37(1):31–34. doi:10.1080/08897077.2015.1132292.
126. White WL, Campbell MD, Shea C, Hoffman HA, Crissman B, Dupont RL. Coparticipation in 12-step mutual aid groups and methadone maintenance treatment: a survey of 322 patients. *J Groups Addict Recover.* 2013; 8(4):294–308. doi:10.1080/1556035X.2013.836872.

127. Monico LB, Gryczynski J, Mitchell SG, et al. Buprenorphine treatment and 12-step meeting attendance: conflicts, compatibilities, and patient outcomes. *J Subst Abus Treat*. 2015;57:89–95. doi:10.1016/j.jsat.2015.05.005.
128. Bentzley BS, Barth KS, Back SE, Book SW. Discontinuation of buprenorphine maintenance therapy: perspectives and outcomes. *J Subst Abuse Treat*. 2015;52:48–57. doi:10.1016/j.jsat.2014.12.011.
129. Gibson A, Degenhardt L, Mattick RP, Ali R, White J, O'Brien S. Exposure to opioid maintenance treatment reduces long-term mortality. *Addiction*. 2008;103(3):462–468. doi:10.1111/j.1360-0443.2007.02090.x.
130. Parran TV, Adelman CA, Merkin B, et al. Long-term outcomes of office-based buprenorphine/naloxone maintenance therapy. *Drug Alcohol Depend*. 2010;106(1):56–60. doi:10.1016/j.drugalcdep.2009.07.013.
131. Fiellin DA, Moore BA, Sullivan LE, et al. Long-term treatment with buprenorphine/naloxone in primary care: results at 2–5 years. *Am J Addict*. 2008;17(2):116–120. doi:10.1080/10550490701860971.
132. Potter JS, Dreifuss JA, Marino EN, et al. The multi-site prescription opioid addiction treatment study: 18-month outcomes. *J Subst Abuse Treat*. 2015;48(1):62–69. doi:10.1016/j.jsat.2014.07.009.
133. Poloméni P, Schwan R. Management of opioid addiction with buprenorphine: French history and current management. *Int J Gen Med*. 2014;7: 143–148. doi:10.2147/IJGM.S53170.
134. White B. Dr. Vincent Dole (1913–2006) on methadone maintenance treatment. *Selected Papers of William L. White*. October 30, 2015. http://www.williamwhitepapers.com/blog/2015/10/dr-vincent-dole-1913-2006-on-methadone-maintenance-treatment.html. Accessed February 27, 2018.
135. Pisani E. Tilting at windmills and the evidence base on injecting drug use. *Lancet*. 2010;376(9737):226–227. doi:10.1016/S0140-6736(10)61132-4.
136. Hawk M, Coulter RWS, Egan JE, et al. Harm reduction principles for healthcare settings. *Harm Reduct J*. 2017;14(70). doi:10.1186/s12954-017-0196-4.
137. Kelly JF, Moos R. Dropout from 12-step self-help groups: prevalence, predictors, and counteracting treatment influences. *J Subst Abuse Treat*. 2003;24(3):241–250. doi:10.1016/S0740-5472(03)00021-7.
138. Kurtz E. *Not-God: A History of Alcoholics Anonymous*. San Francisco, CA: Harper & Row Publishers; 1979.
139. Rathert C, Wyrwich MD, Boren SA. Patient-centered care and outcomes: a systematic review of the literature. *Med Care Res Rev*. 2013;70(4):351–379. doi:10.1177/1077558712465774.
140. Humphreys K, Noke JM. The influence of posttreatment mutual help group participation on the friendship networks of substance abuse patients. *Am J Community Psychol*. 1997;25(1):1–16. doi:10.1023/A:1024613507082.
141. Atkins RG, Hawdon JE. Religiosity and participation in mutual-aid sup-

port groups for addiction. *J Subst Abuse Treat*. 2007;33(3):321–331. doi:10.1016/j.jsat.2007.07.001.

142. Zemore SE, Lui C, Mericle A, Hemberg J, Kaskutas LA. A longitudinal study of the comparative efficacy of Women for Sobriety, LifeRing, SMART Recovery, and 12-step groups for those with AUD. *J Subst Abuse Treat*. 2018;88:18–26. doi:10.1016/j.jsat.2018.02.004.
143. Fenster J. Characteristics of clinicians likely to refer clients to 12-step programs versus a diversity of post-treatment options. *Drug Alcohol Depend*. 2006;83(3):238–246. doi:10.1016/j.drugalcdep.2005.11.017.
144. Kelly JF, White WL. Broadening the base of addiction mutual-help organizations. *J Groups Addict Recover*. 2012;7(2–4):82–101. doi:10.1080/1556035X.2012.705646.
145. Auriacombe M, Denis CM, Beltran V, et al. 10-years outcome of methadone- and buprenorphine-maintained patients: mortality, quality of life and substance use. *Drug Alcohol Depend*. 2014;140:e8. doi:10.1016/j.drugalcdep.2014.02.043.
146. Evans E, Li L, Min J, et al. Mortality among individuals accessing pharmacological treatment for opioid dependence in California, 2006–10. *Addiction*. 2015;110(6):996–1005. doi:10.1111/add.12863.
147. Marsden J, Stillwell G, Jones H, et al. Does exposure to opioid substitution treatment in prison reduce the risk of death after release? A national prospective observational study in England. *Addiction*. 2017;112(8):1408–1418. doi:10.1111/add.13779.
148. Saxon AJ, Hser Y-I, Woody G, Ling W. Medication-assisted treatment for opioid addiction: methadone and buprenorphine. *J Food Drug Anal*. 2013;21(4):S69–S72. doi:10.1016/j.jfda.2013.09.037.
149. Substance Abuse and Mental Health Services Administration. *National Survey of Substance Abuse Treatment Services (N-SSATS): 2016. Data on Substance Abuse Treatment Facilities*. BHSIS Series S-93, HHS Publication No. (SMA) 17-5039. Rockville, MD: SAMHSA; 2017. https://wwwdasis.samhsa.gov/dasis2/nssats/2016_nssats_rpt.pdf. Accessed January 10, 2018.
150. Knudsen HK, Ducharme LJ, Roman PM, Link T. Buprenorphine diffusion: The attitudes of substance abuse treatment counselors. *J Subst Abuse Treat*. 2005;29(2):95–106. doi:10.1016/j.jsat.2005.05.002.
151. Rieckmann T, Daley M, Fuller BE, Thomas CP, McCarty D. Client and counselor attitudes toward the use of medications for treatment of opioid dependence. *J Subst Abuse Treat*. 2007;32(2):207–215. doi:10.1016/j.jsat.2006.09.002.
152. Abraham AJ, Rieckmann T, McNulty T, Kovas AE, Roman PM. Counselor attitudes toward the use of naltrexone in substance abuse treatment: A multi-level modeling approach. *Addict Behav*. 2011;36(6):576–583. doi:10.1016/j.addbeh.2011.01.030.

153. Cunningham CO, Sohler NL, McCoy K, Kunins HV. Attending physicians' and residents' attitudes and beliefs about prescribing buprenorphine at an urban teaching hospital. *Fam Med.* 2006;38(5):336–340. https://fammedarchives.blob.core.windows.net/imagesandpdfs/fmhub/fm2006/May/Chinazo336.pdf. Accessed August 10, 2019.
154. Aletraris L, Edmond MB, Paino M, Fields D, Roman PM. Counselor training and attitudes toward pharmacotherapies for opioid use disorder. *Subst Abus.* 2016;37(1):47–53. doi:10.1080/08897077.2015.1062457.
155. Johnson RA, Lukens JM, Kole JW, Sisti DA. Views about responsibility for alcohol addiction and negative evaluations of naltrexone. *Subst Abuse Treat Prev Policy.* 2015;10(1):10. doi:10.1186/s13011-015-0004-7.
156. Keller DS, Dermatis H. Current status of professional training in the addictions. *Subst Abus.* 1999;20(3):123–140. doi.org/10.1080/08897079909511401.
157. Kerwin ME, Walker-Smith K, Kirby KC. Comparative analysis of state requirements for the training of substance abuse and mental health counselors. *J Subst Abuse Treat.* 2006;30(3):173–181. doi:10.1016/j.jsat.2005.11.004.
158. Mulvey KP, Hubbard S, Hayashi S. A national study of the substance abuse treatment workforce. *J Subst Abus Treat.* 2003;24(1):51–57. doi:10.1016/S0740-5472(02)00322-7.
159. Campbell TC, Catlin LA, Melchert TP. Alcohol and other drug abuse counselors' attitudes and resources for integrating research and practice. *J Drug Educ.* 2003;33(3):307–323. doi:10.2190/VUHN-X36D-KH56-2P77.
160. Wendt DC, Gone JP. Complexities with group therapy facilitation in substance use disorder specialty treatment settings. *J Subst Abuse Treat.* 2018;88:9–17. doi:10.1016/J.JSAT.2018.02.002.
161. *SAMHSA's National Outcome Measure Domains.* https://dhs.iowa.gov/sites/default/files/SAMHSA-National-Outcome-Measures_09-01-2011.pdf. Accessed February 5, 2019.
162. National Association of State Alcohol and Drug Abuse Directors. *State Regulations on Substance Use Disorder Programs and Counselors: An Overview.* Washington, DC: NASADAD; 2012. https://nasadad.org/wp-content/uploads/2010/12/State_Regulation_of_SUD_Programs_and_Counselors-7-26-13.pdf. Updated July 2013. Accessed August 10, 2019.
163. McCarty D, Braude L, Lyman DR, et al. Substance abuse intensive outpatient programs: assessing the evidence. *Psychiatr Serv.* 2014;65(6):718–726. doi:10.1176/appi.ps.201300249.
164. Reif S, George P, Braude L, et al. Residential treatment for individuals with substance use disorders: assessing the evidence. *Psychiatr Serv.* 2014;65(3):301–312. doi:10.1176/appi.ps.201300242.
165. Kourounis G, Richards BD, Kyprianou E, Symeonidou E, Malliori MM,

Samartzis L. Opioid substitution therapy: lowering the treatment thresholds. *Drug Alcohol Depend.* 2016;161:1–8. doi:10.1016/j.drugalcdep.2015.12.021.
166. Carroll KM, Weiss RD. The role of behavioral interventions in buprenorphine maintenance treatment: a review. *Am J Psychiatry.* 2017;174(8):738–747. doi:10.1176/appi.ajp.2016.16070792.
167. Foreman ML, Jefferson T, de La Viez B, et al. *Sharing the Dream: Is the ADA Accommodating All?* Washington, DC: US Commission on Civil Rights; 2000. https://www.usccr.gov/pubs/ada/main.htm. Accessed January 28, 2019.
168. Medication Assisted Treatment for Opioid Use Disorders, 42 CFR §8. https://www.ecfr.gov/cgi-bin/retrieveECFR?gp=&SID=0d945f6e5f6068b536698ccc72159bc8&r=PART&n=42y1.0.1.1.10#se42.1.8_112. Accessed August 10, 2019.
169. Medication-assisted treatment with methadone (MAT) laws [dataset]. Prescription Drug Abuse Policy System website. http://pdaps.org/datasets/medication-assisted-treatment-with-methadone-mat-laws. Published 2016. Accessed August 10, 2019.
170. Dowell D, Haegerich TM, Chou R. CDC guideline for prescribing opioids for chronic pain—United States. *JAMA.* 2016;315(15):1624–1645. doi:10.1001/jama.2016.1464.
171. O'Brien CP, McLellan AT. Myths about the treatment of addiction. *Lancet.* 1996;347(8996):237–240. doi:10.1016/S0140-6736(96)90409-2.
172. Indiana Code 12-23-18-5. http://iga.in.gov/legislative/laws/2019/ic/titles/012#12-23-18-5. Accessed August 10, 2019.
173. Silverman K, Wong CJ, Higgins ST, et al. Increasing opiate abstinence through voucher-based reinforcement therapy. *Drug Alcohol Depend.* 1996;41(2):157–165. doi:10.1016/0376-8716(96)01246-X.
174. Comer SD, Sullivan MA, Vosburg SK, et al. Abuse liability of intravenous buprenorphine/naloxone and buprenorphine alone in buprenorphine-maintained intravenous heroin abusers. *Addiction.* 2010;105(4):709–718. doi:10.1111/j.1360-0443.2009.02843.x.
175. Zhang Z, Friedmann PD, Gerstein DR. Does retention matter? Treatment duration and improvement in drug use. *Addiction.* 2003;98(5):673–684. http://www.ncbi.nlm.nih.gov/pubmed/12751985. Accessed April 26, 2018.
176. Strike C, Millson M, Hopkins S, Smith C. What is low threshold methadone maintenance treatment? *Int J Drug Policy.* 2013;24(6):e51–e56. doi:10.1016/j.drugpo.2013.05.005.
177. Merrill JO, Jackson TR, Schulman BA, et al. Methadone medical maintenance in primary care: an implementation evaluation. *J Gen Intern Med.* 2005;20(4):344–349. doi:10.1111/j.1525-1497.2005.04028.x.
178. Andraka-Christou B, Capone MJ. A qualitative study comparing physician-reported barriers to treating addiction using buprenorphine

and extended-release naltrexone in US office-based practices. *Int J Drug Policy*. 2018;54:9–17. doi:10.1016/j.drugpo.2017.11.021.

179. Addiction medicine. American Board of Preventive Medicine website. http://www.theabpm.org/become-certified/subspecialties/addiction-medicine. Accessed June 3, 2018.

180. Alderks CE. *The CBHSQ Report: Trends in the Use of Methadone, Buprenorphine, and Extended-Release Naltrexone at Substance Abuse Treatment Facilities: 2003–2015 (Update)*. Rockville, MD: Center for Behavioral Health Statistics and Quality, Substance Abuse and Mental Health Services Administration; 2017. https://www.samhsa.gov/data/sites/default/files/report_3192/ShortReport-3192.pdf. Accessed January 23, 2018.

181. Joseph H, Stancliff S, Langrod J. Methadone maintenance treatment (MMT): a review of historical and clinical issues. *Mt Sinai J Med*. 2000; 67(5–6):347–364. PMID:11064485.

182. D'Aunno T, Pollack HA, Frimpong JA, Wuchiett D. Evidence-based treatment for opioid disorders: a 23-year national study of methadone dose levels. *J Subst Abuse Treat*. 2014;47(4):245–250. doi:10.1016/j.jsat.2014.06.001.

183. Johnson RE, Chutuape M, Strain EC, Walsh SL, Stitzer ML, Bigelow GE. A comparison of levomethadyl acetate, buprenorphine, and methadone for opioid dependence. *N Engl J Med*. 2000;343(18):1290–1297. doi:10.1056/NEJM200011023431802.

184. Strain E, Bigelow GE, Liebson I, Stitzer ML. Moderate- vs high-dose methadone in the treatment of opioid dependence: a randomized trial. *JAMA*. 1999;281(11):1000–1005. doi:10.1001/jama.281.11.1000.

185. Strain EC. Methadone dose during maintenance treatment. In: Strain EC, Stitzer ML, eds. *The Treatment of Opioid Dependence*. Baltimore, MD: Johns Hopkins University Press; 2006:89–118.

186. Donny EC, Walsh SL, Bigelow GE, Eissenberg T, Stitzer ML. High-dose methadone produces superior opioid blockade and comparable withdrawal suppression to lower doses in opioid-dependent humans. *Psychopharmacology (Berl)*. 2002;161(2):202–212. doi:10.1007/s00213-002-1027-0.

187. Bakalar N. Vital signs patterns: many fatal overdoses linked to methadone. *Well* (blog). *New York Times*. July 9, 2012. https://well.blogs.nytimes.com/2012/07/09/many-fatal-overdoses-linked-to-methadone. Accessed August 10, 2019.

188. Duffy P, Baldwin H. The nature of methadone diversion in England: a Merseyside case study. *Harm Reduct J*. 2012;9(1):3. doi:10.1186/1477-7517-9-3.

189. Johnson B, Richert T. Diversion of methadone and buprenorphine from opioid substitution treatment: the importance of patients' attitudes and norms. *J Subst Abuse Treat*. 2015;54:50–55. doi:10.1016/j.jsat.2015.01.013.

190. Harris M, Rhodes T. Methadone diversion as a protective strategy: The harm reduction potential of "generous constraints." *Int J Drug Policy*. 2013;24(6):e43–e50. doi:10.1016/j.drugpo.2012.10.003.
191. Barnett PG, Zaric GS, Brandeau ML. The cost-effectiveness of buprenorphine maintenance therapy for opiate addiction in the United States. *Addiction*. 2001;96(9):1267–1278. doi:10.1080/09652140120070328.
192. Byford S, Barrett B, Metrebian N, et al. Cost-effectiveness of injectable opioid treatment v. oral methadone for chronic heroin addiction. *Br J Psychiatry*. 2013;203(5):341–349. doi:10.1192/bjp.bp.112.111583.
193. Tolia VN, Murthy K, Bennett MM, et al. Morphine vs methadone treatment for infants with neonatal abstinence syndrome. *J Pediatr*. 2018;203: 185–189. doi:10.1016/j.jpeds.2018.07.061.
194. Young JL, Martin PR. Treatment of opioid dependence in the setting of pregnancy. *Psychiatr Clin North Am*. 2012;35(2):441–460. doi:10.1016/j.psc.2012.03.008.
195. Wilder CM, Winhusen T. Pharmacological management of opioid use disorder in pregnant women. *CNS Drugs*. 2015;29(8):625–636. doi:10.1007/s40263-015-0273-8.
196. Substance Abuse and Mental Health Services Administration. *Federal Guidelines for Opioid Treatment Programs*. HHS Publication No. (SMA) PEP15-FEDGUIDEOTP. Rockville, MD: SAMHSA; 2015. https://store.samhsa.gov/system/files/pep15-fedguideotp.pdf. Accessed August 10, 2019.
197. Amato L, Minozzi S, Vecchi S, Davoli M, Perucci CA. An overview of Cochrane systematic reviews of pharmacological and psychosocial treatment of opioid dependence. Background paper for the meeting "1st Consultation on Technical Guidelines for Treatment of Opioid Dependence." Geneva, Switzerland: World Health Organization; November, 1–4, 2005. https://www.who.int/substance_abuse/activities/overview_of_cochrane_systematic_reviews.pdf. Accessed August 10, 2019.
198. World Health Organization. *Guidelines for the Psychosocially Assisted Pharmacological Treatment of Opioid Dependence*. Geneva, Switzerland: WHO; 2009. https://www.who.int/substance_abuse/publications/opioid_dependence_guidelines.pdf. Accessed August 10, 2019.
199. Andrilla CHA, Moore TE, Patterson DG, Larson EH. Geographic distribution of providers with a DEA waiver to prescribe buprenorphine for the treatment of opioid use disorder: a 5-year update. *J Rural Heal*. 2019;35(1): 108–112. doi:10.1111/jrh.12307.
200. Ghertner R. U.S. trends in the supply of providers with a waiver to prescribe buprenorphine for opioid use disorder in 2016 and 2018. *Drug Alcohol Depend*. 2019;204(1):107527. doi:10.1016/j.drugalcdep.2019.06.029.

201. Sigmon SC. The untapped potential of office-based buprenorphine treatment. *JAMA Psychiatry*. 2015;72(4):395–396. doi:10.1001/jamapsychiatry.2014.2421.
202. Jones CM, Campopiano M, Baldwin G, McCance-Katz E. National and state treatment need and capacity for opioid agonist medication-assisted treatment. *Am J Public Health*. 2015;105(8):e55–e63. doi:10.2105/AJPH.2015.302664.
203. Thomas CP, Doyle E, Kreiner PW, et al. Prescribing patterns of buprenorphine waivered physicians. *Drug Alcohol Depend*. 2017;181:213–218. doi:10.1016/j.drugalcdep.2017.10.002.
204. National Institute on Drug Abuse. *Drugs, Brains, and Behavior: The Science of Addiction*. NIH Publication No. 18-DA-5605. Washington, DC: National Institues of Health; 2007. https://d14rmgtrwzf5a.cloudfront.net/sites/default/files/soa.pdf. Revised 2008, 2010, 2014, 2018. Accessed October 27, 2018.
205. Midmer D, Kahan M, Wilson L. Medical students' experiences with addicted patients: a web-based survey. *Subst Abus*. 2008;29(1):25–32. doi:10.1300/J465v29n01_04.
206. American Society of Addiction Medicine. *Public Policy Statement on the Addiction Medicine Physician Participation in and Leadership of Multidisciplinary Care Teams*. Chevy Chase, MD: ASAM; 2016. https://www.asam.org/docs/default-source/public-policy-statements/multidisciplinary-care-teams-final-jan-2016.pdf. Accessed January 16, 2019.
207. Vestal C. Nurse licensing laws block treatment for opioid addiction. *Stateline*, an initiative of The Pew Charitable Trusts. April 21, 2017. http://www.pewtrusts.org/en/research-and-analysis/blogs/stateline/2017/04/21/nurse-licensing-laws-block-treatment-for-opioid-addiction. Accessed August 10, 2019.
208. Polydorou S, Gunderson EW, Levin FR. Training physicians to treat substance use disorders. *Curr Psychiatry Rep*. 2008;10(5):399–404. doi:10.1007/s11920-008-0064-8.
209. Wakeman SE, Baggett M V, Pham-Kanter G, Campbell EG. Internal medicine residents' training in substance use disorders: a survey of the quality of instruction and residents' self-perceived preparedness to diagnose and treat addiction. *Subst Abus*. 2013;34(4):363–370. doi:10.1080/08897077.2013.797540.
210. Yoast RA, Filstead WJ, Wilford BB, Hayashi S, Reenan J, Epstein J. Teaching about substance abuse. *Virtual Mentor*. 2008;10(1):21–29. doi:10.1001/virtualmentor.2008.10.1.medu1-0801.
211. Grant BF, Saha TD, Ruan WJ, et al. Epidemiology of *DSM-5* drug use disorder: results from the National Epidemiologic Survey on Alcohol and Related Conditions-III. *JAMA Psychiatry*. 2016;73(1):39–47. doi:10.1001/jamapsychiatry.2015.2132.

212. Gunderson EW, Fiellin DA, Levin FR, Sullivan LE, Kleber HD. Evaluation of a combined online and in person training in the use of buprenorphine. *Subst Abus*. 2006;27(3):39–45. doi:10.1300/J465v27n03_06.
213. Weber EM. Failure of physicians to prescribe pharmacotherapies for addiction: regulatory restrictions and physician resistance. *J Health Care L & Pol'y*. 2010;13(1):49–76. https://pdfs.semanticscholar.org/da98/9a10 3ed577a89a4e76d03242bd617759d0bb.pdf. Accessed August 10, 2019.
214. Voon P, Karamouzian M, Kerr T. Chronic pain and opioid misuse: a review of reviews. *Subst Abuse Treat Prev Policy*. 2017;12(1):36. doi:10.1186 /s13011-017-0120-7.
215. Ross S, Peselow E. Co-occurring psychotic and addictive disorders: neurobiology and diagnosis. *Clin Neuropharmacol*. 2012;35(5):235–243. doi:10.1097/WNF.0b013e318261e193.
216. Tanner TB, Wilhelm SE, Rossie KM, Metcalf MP. Web-based SBIRT skills training for health professional students and primary care providers. *Subst Abus*. 2012;33(3):316–320. doi:10.1080/08897077.2011.640151.
217. Egan JE, Casadonte P, Gartenmann T, et al. The Physician Clinical Support System–Buprenorphine (PCSS-B): a novel project to expand/ improve buprenorphine treatment. *J Gen Intern Med*. 2010;25(9):936–941. doi:10.1007/s11606-010-1377-y.
218. Harris AHS, Bowe T, Hagedorn H, et al. Multifaceted academic detailing program to increase pharmacotherapy for alcohol use disorder: interrupted time series evaluation of effectiveness. *Addict Sci Clin Pract*. 2016; 11(1):15. doi:10.1186/s13722-016-0063-8.
219. Stein BD, Pacula RL, Gordon AJ, et al. Where is buprenorphine dispensed to treat opioid use disorders? The role of private offices, opioid treatment programs, and substance abuse treatment facilities in urban and rural counties. *Milbank Q*. 2015;93(3):561–583. doi:10.1111/1468-0009.12137.
220. Sullivan LE, Fiellin DA. Office-based buprenorphine for patients with opioid dependence. *Ann Intern Med*. 2008;148(9):662–670. https://www .ncbi.nlm.nih.gov/pmc/articles/PMC3694223/. Accessed August 10, 2019.
221. McCarty D, Rieckmann T, Baker RL, McConnell KJ. The perceived impact of 42 CFR Part 2 on coordination and integration of care: a qualitative analysis. *Psychiatr Serv*. 2017;68(3):245–249. doi:10.1176/appi.ps .201600138.
222. Uses and disclosures to carry out treatment, payment, or health care operations, 45 CFR §164.506(c)(2).
223. Permitted uses and disclosures: exchange for treatment [fact sheet]. Washington, DC: Office of the National Coordinator for Health Information Technology and Office for Civil Rights, US Department of Health and Human Services; January 2016. https://www.hhs.gov/sites/default /files/exchange_treatment.pdf. Accessed October 23, 2018.

224. Final rule: 42 CFR Part 2, confidentiality of substance use disorder patient records. American Psychiatric Association website. https://www.psychiatry.org/psychiatrists/practice/practice-management/hipaa/42-cfr-part-2. Accessed August 10, 2019.
225. D'Onofrio G, Chawarski MC, O'Connor PG, et al. Emergency department–initiated buprenorphine for opioid dependence with continuation in primary care: outcomes during and after intervention. *J Gen Intern Med.* 2017;32(6):660–666. doi:10.1007/s11606-017-3993-2.
226. Liebschutz JM, Crooks D, Herman D, et al. Buprenorphine treatment for hospitalized, opioid-dependent patients: a randomized clinical trial. *JAMA Intern Med.* 2014;174(8):1369–1376. doi:10.1001/jamainternmed.2014.2556.
227. Administering or dispensing of narcotic drugs, 21 CFR §1306.07(b).
228. Huhn AS, Dunn KE. Why aren't physicians prescribing more buprenorphine? *J Subst Abuse Treat.* 2017;78:1–7. doi:10.1016/j.jsat.2017.04.005.
229. Saxon AJ, McCarty D. Challenges in the adoption of new pharmacotherapeutics for addiction to alcohol and other drugs. *Pharmacol Ther.* 2005;108(1):119–128. doi:10.1016/j.pharmthera.2005.06.014.
230. Hutchinson E, Catlin M, Andrilla CH, Baldwin LM, Rosenblatt RA. Barriers to primary care physicians prescribing buprenorphine. *Ann Fam Med.* 2014;12(2):128–133. doi:10.1370/afm.1595.
231. Furst RT. Diffusion and diversion of suboxone: an exploration of illicit street opioid selling. *J Addict Dis.* 2014;33(3):177–186. doi:10.1080/10550887.2014.950030.
232. Lofwall MR, Walsh SL. A review of buprenorphine diversion and misuse: the current evidence base and experiences from around the world. *J Addict Med.* 2014;8(5):315–326. doi:10.1097/ADM.0000000000000045.
233. Kissin W, McLeod C, Sonnefeld J, Stanton A. Experiences of a national sample of qualified addiction specialists who have and have not prescribed buprenorphine for opioid dependence. *J Addict Dis.* 2006;25(4):91–103. doi:10.1300/J069v25n04_09.
234. Alderks CE. Trends in the use of methadone and buprenorphine at substance abuse treatment facilities: 2003 to 2011. In: *The CBHSQ Report.* Rockville, MD: Center for Behavioral Health Statistics and Quality, Substance Abuse and Mental Health Services Administration; 2013. https://www.ncbi.nlm.nih.gov/books/NBK384659. Accessed August 10, 2019.
235. Knudsen HK, Abraham AJ, Roman PM. Adoption and implementation of medications in addiction treatment programs. *J Addict Med.* 2011;5(1):21–27. doi:10.1097/ADM.0b013e3181d41ddb.
236. Ducharme LJ, Knudsen HK, Roman PM, Johnson JA. Innovation adoption in substance abuse treatment: exposure, trialability, and the Clinical Trials Network. *J Subst Abuse Treat.* 2007;32(4):321–329. doi:10.1016/j.jsat.2006.05.021.

237. Rieckmann T, Abraham A, Zwick J, Rasplica C, McCarty D. A longitudinal study of state strategies and policies to accelerate evidence-based practices in the context of systems transformation. *Health Serv Res*. 2015; 50(4):1125–1145. doi:10.1111/1475-6773.12273.
238. Substance Abuse and Mental Health Services Administration. *Medicaid Handbook: Interface with Behavioral Health Services*. HHS Publication No. SMA-13-4773. Rockville, MD: Substance Abuse and Mental Health Services Administration, 2013. https://store.samhsa.gov/system/files/sma13-4773_mod7.pdf Accessed September 17, 2018.
239. Kermack A, Flannery M, Tofighi B, McNeely J, Lee JD. Buprenorphine prescribing practice trends and attitudes among New York providers. *J Subst Abuse Treat*. 2017;74:1–6. doi:10.1016/j.jsat.2016.10.005.
240. Clark RE, Baxter JD, Barton BA, Aweh G, O'Connell E, Fisher WH. The impact of prior authorization on buprenorphine dose, relapse rates, and cost for Massachusetts Medicaid beneficiaries with opioid dependence. *Health Serv Res*. 2014;49(6):1964–1979. doi:10.1111/1475-6773.12201.
241. Mark TL, Lubran R, McCance-Katz EF, Chalk M, Richardson J. Medicaid coverage of medications to treat alcohol and opioid dependence. *J Subst Abuse Treat*. 2015;55:1–5. doi:10.1016/j.jsat.2015.04.009.
242. Reif S, Horgan CM, Hodgkin D, Matteucci AM, Creedon TB, Stewart MT. Access to addiction pharmacotherapy in private health plans. *J Subst Abus Treat*. 2016;66:23–29. doi:10.1016/j.jsat.2016.03.001.
243. Becerra, X. Prior authorization requirements for medication-assisted treatment of opioid use disorder [letter]. February 14, 2019. Sacramento: State of California, Office of the Attorney General. https://oag.ca.gov/system/files/attachments/press-docs/matletter.pdf. Accessed August 10, 2019.
244. McAneny B. Landmark deal on medication-assisted treatment a model for nation. *Leadership Viewpoints*. American Medical Association (AMA) website. January 7, 2019. https://www.ama-assn.org/advocacy/leadership-viewpoints/landmark-deal-medication-assisted-treatment-model-nation. Accessed January 16, 2019.
245. Clark RE, Samnaliev M, Baxter JD, Leung GY. The evidence doesn't justify steps by state Medicaid programs to restrict opioid addiction treatment with buprenorphine. *Health Aff (Millwood)*. 2011;30(8):1425–1433. doi:10.1377/hlthaff.2010.0532.
246. Behavioral health services. *Medicaid.gov*. Centers for Medicare and Medicaid Services. https://www.medicaid.gov/medicaid/benefits/bhs/index.html. Accessed September 17, 2018.
247. Bowling B, Newman D, White C, Wood A, Coustasse A. Provider reimbursement following the Affordable Care Act. Paper presented at: Business and Health Administration Association Annual Conference; March

22–24, 2017; Chicago, IL. http://mds.marshall.edu/mgmt_faculty/174. Accessed August 10, 2019.

248. *The Psychiatric Shortage: Causes and Solutions*. Washington, DC: National Council Medical Director Institute; 2017. https://www.thenational council.org/wp-content/uploads/2017/03/Psychiatric-Shortage _National-Council-.pdf. Accessed August 10, 2019.

249. Hinde J, Hayes J, Mark T, Bernstein S, Karon SL. *State and Local Policy Levers for Increasing Treatment and Recovery Capacity to Address the Opioid Epidemic: Final Report*. Washington, DC: Office of the Assistant Secretary for Planning and Evaluation, US Department of Health and Human Services; 2017. https://aspe.hhs.gov/basic-report/state-and-local-policy -levers-increasing-treatment-and-recovery-capacity-address-opioid -epidemic-final-report. Accessed August 10, 2019.

250. Drug courts [fact sheet]. Washington, DC: US Department of Justice, Office of Justice Programs; May 2018. https://www.ncjrs.gov/pdffiles1 /nij/238527.pdf. Accessed July 11, 2018.

251. Supreme Court of the State of Florida. *Florida Adult Drug Court Best Practice Standards*. Tallahassee, FL: Florida State Courts; 2017. https://www .flcourts.org/content/download/217042/1968198/Florida_Adult_Drug _Court_Standards_I-X.pdf. Accessed May 29, 2019.

252. National Association of Drug Court Professionals' Drug Court Standards Committee. *Defining Drug Courts: The Key Components*. Drug Courts Resource Series. Washington, DC: Bureau of Justice Assistance; 2004. https://www.ncjrs.gov/pdffiles1/bja/205621.pdf. Accessed May 29, 2019.

253. Public policy statement on medical ethics with annotations applicable to addiction medicine background. Rockville, MD: American Society of Addiction Medicine; January 23, 2019. https://www.asam.org/docs /default-source/public-policy-statements/public-policy-statement-on -medical-ethicsa98c289472bc604ca5b7ff000030b21a.pdf. Accessed February 20, 2019.

254. IL Staff. AG touts benefits of incarcerating drug offenders to help end cycle of addiction. *Indiana Lawyer*. June 9, 2017. https://www.theindiana lawyer.com/articles/43943-ag-touts-benefits-of-incarcerating-drug -offenders-to-help-end-cycle-of-addiction. Accessed August 10, 2019.

255. Ettner SL, Huang D, Evans E, et al. Benefit-cost in the California treatment outcome project: does substance abuse treatment "pay for itself"? *Health Serv Res*. 2006;41(1):192–213. doi:10.1111/j.1475-6773.2005 .00466.x.

256. Marlowe DB. Integrating substance abuse treatment and criminal justice supervision. *Sci Pract Perspect*. 2003;2(1):4–14. http://www.ncbi.nlm.nih .gov/pubmed/18552716. Accessed August 5, 2018.

257. Green TC, Clarke J, Brinkley-Rubinstein L, et al. Postincarceration fatal overdoses after implementing medications for addiction treatment in a

statewide correctional system. *JAMA Psychiatry*. 2018;75(4):405–407. doi:10.1001/jamapsychiatry.2017.4614.

258. Nunn A, Zaller N, Dickman S, Trimbur C, Nijhawan A, Rich JD. Methadone and buprenorphine prescribing and referral practices in US prison systems: results from a nationwide survey. *Drug Alcohol Depend*. 2009; 105(1–2):83–88. doi:10.1016/j.drugalcdep.2009.06.015.
259. Moore KE, Roberts W, Reid HH, Smith KMZ, Oberleitner LMS, McKee SA. Effectiveness of medication assisted treatment for opioid use in prison and jail settings: a meta-analysis and systematic review. *J Subst Abuse Treat*. 2019;99:32–43. doi:10.1016/j.jsat.2018.12.003.
260. Hora PF, Stalcup T. Drug treatment courts in the twenty-first century: the evolution of the revolution in problem-solving courts. *Georgia Law Rev*. 2008;42:717–811. http://ndcrc.org/wp-content/uploads/2017/05/hora-stalcup.pdf. Accessed August 10, 2019.
261. Miller EJ. Embracing addiction: drug courts and the false promise of judicial interventionism. *Ohio State Law J*. 2004;65:1479–1576. https://pdfs.semanticscholar.org/e302/c28c46fbf0f738fa30a604dc0b7c7d61d965.pdf. Accessed August 10, 2019.
262. Matusow H, Dickman SL, Rich JD, et al. Medication assisted treatment in US drug courts: results from a nationwide survey of availability, barriers, and attitudes. *J Subst Abuse Treat*. 2013;44(5):473–480. doi:10.1016/j.jsat.2012.10.004.
263. Krawczyk N, Picher CE, Feder KA, Saloner B. Only one in twenty justice-referred adults in specialty treatment for opioid use receive methadone or buprenorphine. *Health Aff (Millwood)*. 2017;36(12):2046–2053. doi:10.1377/hlthaff.2017.0890.
264. Monico LB, Mitchell SG, Gryczynski J, et al. Prior experience with non-prescribed buprenorphine: role in treatment entry and retention. *J Subst Abuse Treat*. 2015;57:57–62. doi:10.1016/j.jsat.2015.04.010.
265. Lofwall MR, Havens JR. Inability to access buprenorphine treatment as a risk factor for using diverted buprenorphine. *Drug Alcohol Depend*. 2012; 126(3):379–383. doi:10.1016/j.drugalcdep.2012.05.025.
266. Carroll JJ, Rich JD, Green TC. The more things change: buprenorphine/naloxone diversion continues while treatment remains inaccessible. *J Addict Med*. 2018;12(6):459–465. doi:10.1097/ADM.0000000000000436.
267. Stöver H. Barriers to opioid substitution treatment access, entry, and retention: a survey of opioid users, patients in treatment, and treating and non-treating physicians. *Eur Addict Res*. 2011;17(1):44–54. doi:10.1159/000320576.
268. Gallas EM. Endorsing religion: drug courts and the 12-step recovery support program. *Am Univ Law Rev*. 2004;53(5):1063–1101. http://digitalcommons.wcl.american.edu/aulr/vol53/iss5/3. Accessed August 10, 2019.

269. Nordstrom BR, Marlowe DB. *Medication-Assisted Treatment for Opioid Use Disorders in Drug Courts*. Alexandria, VA: National Drug Court Institute; 2016. Drug Court Practioner Fact Sheet 11(2). https://www.ndci.org/wp-content/uploads/2019/01/mat_fact_sheet-1.pdf. Accessed July 16, 2018.
270. *Smith v Aroostook County*, Docket No. 1:18-cv-352-NT (D. Me. 2019), aff'd, No. 19-1340, (1st Cir. 2019). https://ecf.med.uscourts.gov/docpub/09102401220. Accessed August 10, 2019.
271. Eickelberg C. Probation officers should never direct medical care for people with OUD. *Filter Magazine*. June 6, 2019. https://filtermag.org/2019/06/06/probation-officers-should-never-direct-medical-care-for-people-with-oud/amp. Accessed August 10, 2019.
272. An act relating to drug treatment, SB 910, 80th Leg Assem, Reg Sess, (Or 2019). https://olis.leg.state.or.us/liz/2019R1/Downloads/MeasureDocument/SB910/Enrolled. Accessed June 18, 2019.
273. Andraka-Christou B, Gabriel M, Madeira J, Silverman RD. Court personnel attitudes towards medications for opioid use disorder: a statewide survey. *J. Subst Abuse Treat*. 2019;104:72–82. doi:10.1016/j.jsat.2019.06.011.
274. Davies J. White House takes important first step toward fixing broken drug court system. *Drug Policy Alliance Blog*. February 5, 2015. http://www.drugpolicy.org/blog/white-house-takes-important-first-step-toward-fixing-broken-drug-court-system. Accessed August 10, 2019.
275. Allen RS, Olson BD. Predicting attrition in the treatment of substance use disorders. *Int J Ment Health Addict*. 2016;14(5):728–742. https://link.springer.com/article/10.1007/s11469-015-9602-x. Accessed August 10, 2019.
276. Patient Protection and Affordable Care Act of 2010, Pub L No. 111-148, 124 Stat 119.
277. Kresina TF. Medication assisted treatment of drug abuse and dependence: global availability and utilization. *Recent Pat Antiinfect Drug Discov*. 2007; 2(1):79–86. doi:10.2174/157489107779561652.
278. Ysa T, Colom J, Abareda A, Ramon A, Carrion M, Segura L. *Governance of Addictions: European Public Policies*. Oxford, UK: Oxford University Press; 2014.
279. Chatwin C. Multi-level governance: the way forward for European illicit drug policy? *Int J Drug Policy*. 2007;18(6):494–502. doi:10.1016/j.drugpo.2006.12.005.
280. Best practice portal. European Monitoring Centre for Drugs and Drug Addiction website. http://www.emcdda.europa.eu/best-practice_en. Accessed September 20, 2018.
281. Laqueur H. Uses and abuses of drug decriminalization in Portugal. *Law Soc Inq*. 2015;40(3):746–781. doi:10.1111/lsi.12104.

282. Portugal Law 15/93 of January 22, 1993, Chapter IV, Article 40–41.
283. Portugal Law 30/2000 of November 29, 2000, Art 2. (Entered into force July 2001).
284. Nagin DS. Deterrence in the twenty-first century. *Crime and Justice*. 2013; 42(1):199–263. doi:10.1086/670398.
285. National Institute of Justice. Five things about deterrence [fact sheet]. NCJ 247350. Washginton, DC: US Department of Justice, Office of Justice Programs; 2016. https://www.ncjrs.gov/pdffiles1/nij/247350.pdf. Accessed August 10, 2019.
286. Messaadi N, Pansu A, Cohen O, Cottencin O. Pharmacists' role in the continued care of patients under opiate substitution treatment. *Therapie*. 2013;68(6):393–400. doi:10.2515/therapie/2013059.
287. Guillou Landreat M, Rozaire C, Guillet JY, Victorri Vigneau C, Le Reste JY, Grall Bronnec M. French experience with buprenorphine: do physicians follow the guidelines? *PLoS One*. 2015;10(10):e0137708. doi:10.1371/journal.pone.0137708.
288. Feroni I, Peretti-Watel P, Masut A, Coudert C, Paraponaris A, Obadia Y. French general practitioners' prescribing high-dosage buprenorphine maintenance treatment: is the existing training (good) enough? *Addict Behav*. 2005;30(1):187–191. doi:10.1016/j.addbeh.2004.04.019.
289. Moatti JP, Souville M, Escaffre N, Obadia Y. French general practitioners' attitudes toward maintenance drug abuse treatment with buprenorphine. *Addiction*. 1998;93(10):1567–1575. PMID:9926562.
290. Auriacombe M, Fatséas M, Dubernet J, Daulouède J-P, Tignol J. French field experience with buprenorphine. *Am J Addict*. 2004;13(S1):S17–S28. doi:10.1080=10550490490440780.
291. Jeantaud I, Harambaru F, Begaud B. Substitution treatment for opiate dependence: survey of community pharmacies in Aquitaine. *Therapie*. 1999;54(2):251–255.
292. Feroni I, Aubisson S, Bouhik A, et al. Collaboration between general practitioners and pharmacists in the management of patients on high-dosage buprenorphine treatment. *Press Med*. 2005;34(17):1213–1219.
293. Idrisov B, Murphy SM, Morrill T, Saadoun M, Lunze K, Shepard D. Implementation of methadone therapy for opioid use disorder in Russia: a modeled cost-effectiveness analysis. *Subst Abuse Treat Prev Policy*. 2017; 12(1):4. doi:10.1186/s13011-016-0087-9.
294. Altice FL, Azbel L, Stone J, et al. The perfect storm: incarceration and the high-risk environment perpetuating transmission of HIV, hepatitis C virus, and tuberculosis in Eastern Europe and Central Asia. *Lancet*. 2016; 388(10050):1228–1248. doi:10.1016/S0140-6736(16)30856-X.
295. Bobrova N, Alcorn R, Rhodes T, Rughnikov I, Neifeld E, Power R. Injection drug users' perceptions of drug treatment services and attitudes toward substitution therapy: a qualitative study in three Russian cities.

J Subst Abuse Treat. 2007;33(4):373–378. doi:10.1016/j.jsat.2007.02.002.

296. MacArthur GJ, Minozzi S, Martin N, et al. Opiate substitution treatment and HIV transmission in people who inject drugs: systematic review and meta-analysis. *BMJ*. 2012;345:e5945. doi:10.1136/bmj.e5945.
297. Elovich R, Drucker E. On drug treatment and social control: Russian narcology's great leap backwards. *Harm Reduct J*. 2008;5(1):23. doi:10.1186/1477-7517-5-23.
298. Bachireddy C, Soule MC, Izenberg JM, Dvoryak S, Dumchev K, Altice F. Integration of health services improves multiple healthcare outcomes among HIV-infected people who inject drugs in Ukraine. *Drug Alcohol Depend*. 2014;134:106–114. doi:10.1016/j.drugalcdep.2013.09.020.
299. Lawrinson P, Ali R, Buavirat A, et al. Key findings from the WHO collaborative study on substitution therapy for opioid dependence and HIV/AIDS. *Addiction*. 2008;103(9):1484–1492. doi:10.1111/j.1360-0443.2008.02249.x.
300. Holt E. Fears over future of opioid substitution therapy in Crimea. *Lancet*. 2014;383(9923):1113. doi:10.1016/S0140-6736(14)60234-8.
301. World Health Organization. *ATLAS of Substance Use Disorders: Resources for the Prevention and Treatment of Substance Use Disorders, Russian Federation*. Geneva, Switzerland: WHO; 2010. http://www.who.int/substance_abuse/publications/atlas_report/profiles/russian_federation.pdf. Accessed October 11, 2018.
302. McKeganey N, Russell C, Cockayne L. Medically assisted recovery from opiate dependence within the context of the UK drug strategy: methadone and Suboxone (buprenorphine-naloxone) patients compared. *J Subst Abuse Treat*. 2013;44(1):97–102. doi:10.1016/j.jsat.2012.04.003.
303. Strang J, Sheridan J, Hunt C, Kerr B, Gerada C, Pringle M. The prescribing of methadone and other opioids to addicts: national survey of GPs in England and Wales. *Br J Gen Pract*. 2005;55(515):444–451.
304. Chutuape MA, Silverman K, Stitzer ML. Survey assessment of methadone treatment services as reinforcers. *Am J Drug Alcohol Abuse*. 1998;24(1):1–16. doi:10.3109/00952999809001695.
305. Clinical Guidelines on Drug Misuse and Dependence Update 2017 Independent Expert Working Group. *Drug Misuse and Dependence: UK Guidelines on Clinical Management*. London, England: Department of Health; 2017. https://assets.publishing.service.gov.uk/government/uploads/system/uploads/attachment_data/file/673978/clinical_guidelines_2017.pdf. Accessed August 10, 2019.
306. Strang J, Manning V, Mayet S, Ridge G, Best D, Sheridan J. Does prescribing for opiate addiction change after national guidelines? Methadone and buprenorphine prescribing to opiate addicts by general practitioners and hospital doctors in England, 1995–2005. *Addiction*. 2007;102(5):761–770. doi:10.1111/j.1360-0443.2007.01762.x.

307. Harper, J. Price's remarks on opioid treatment were unscientific and damaging, experts say. *Shots: Health News from NPR*. National Public Radio. May 16, 2017. https://www.npr.org/sections/health-shots/2017/05/16/528614422/prices-remarks-on-opioid-treatment-were-unscientific-and-damaging-experts-say. Accessed August 10, 2019.
308. Duke K. Exchanging expertise and constructing boundaries: the development of a transnational knowledge network around heroin-assisted treatment. *Int J Drug Policy*. 2016;31:56–63. doi:10.1016/j.drugpo.2015.12.004.
309. Strang J, Groshkova T, Metrebian N. *New Heroin-Assisted Treatment: Recent Evidence and Current Practices of Supervised Injectable Heroin Treatment in Europe and Beyond*. Luxembourg: European Monitoring Centre for Drugs and Drug Addiction; 2012. doi:10.2810/50141.
310. Csete J, Kamarulzaman A, Kazatchkine M, et al. Public health and international drug policy. *Lancet*. 2016;387(10026):1427–1480. doi:10.1016/S0140-6736(16)00619-X.
311. Heroin assisted treatment (HAT): saving lives, improving health, reducing crime [briefing]. Bristol, England: Transform Drug Policy Foundation; 2017. https://transformdrugs.org/wp-content/uploads/2018/10/HAT-Briefing-2017.pdf. Accessed January 31, 2019.
312. Marshall BD, Milloy M-J, Wood E, Montaner JS, Kerr T. Reduction in overdose mortality after the opening of North America's first medically supervised safer injecting facility: a retrospective population-based study. *Lancet*. 2011;377(9775):1429–1437. doi:10.1016/S0140-6736(10)62353-7.
313. Lawrence TB. High-stakes institutional translation: establishing North America's first government-sanctioned supervised injection site. *Acad Manag J*. 2017;60(5):1771–1800. doi:10.5465/amj.2015.0714.
314. National Institute of Medicine. *Crossing the Quality Chasm: A New Health System for the 21st Century*. Washington DC: National Academies Press; 2001. doi:10.17226/10027.
315. Gerteis M, Edgman-Levitan S, Daley J, Delbanco TL, eds. *Through the Patient's Eyes: Understanding and Promoting Person-Centered Care*. San Fransisco, CA: John Wiley & Sons Ltd; 1993.
316. Dreifuss JA, Griffin ML, Frost K, et al. Patient characteristics associated with buprenorphine/naloxone treatment outcome for prescription opioid dependence: results from a multisite study. *Drug Alcohol Depend*. 2013;131(1–2):112–118. doi:10.1016/j.drugalcdep.2012.12.010.
317. Weiss RD, Griffin ML, Potter JS, et al. Who benefits from additional drug counseling among prescription opioid-dependent patients receiving buprenorphine-naloxone and standard medical management? *Drug Alcohol Depend*. 2014;140:118–122. doi:10.1016/j.drugalcdep.2014.04.005.

Index